Rheumatology

Questions and Answers

EDITOR/AUTHOR:

HAROLD M ADELMAN, MD, FACP, FACR
Professor of Medicine, Division of Rheumatology, University of South Florida Health Sciences Center and Director, Residents' Internal Medicine Clinic, James A. Haley Veterans' Hospital

AUTHORS:

JOHN D CARTER, MD, FACR
Assistant Professor of Medicine, Division of Rheumatology University of South Florida Health Sciences Center

JOANNE VALERIANO-MARCET, MD, FACR
Associate Professor of Medicine, Division of Rheumatology University of South Florida Health Sciences Center

KEITH S KANIK, MD, FACR
Assistant Professor of Medicine, Division of Rheumatology University of South Florida Health Sciences Center

MITCHEL J SELEZNICK, MD, FACP, FACR
Associate Professor of Medicine, Division of General Medicine University of South Florida Health Sciences Center

BRYAN A BOGNAR, MD, FACP
Associate Professor of Medicine, Division of General Medicine Interim Dean for Educational Affairs, University of South Florida Health Sciences Center

EDWARD P CUTOLO, MD
Associate Professor of Medicine, Division of General Medicine University of South Florida Health Sciences Center and Chief of Staff, James A. Haley Veterans' Hospital

RAJANI P SHAH, MD
Assistant Professor of Medicine, Division of General Medicine University of South Florida Health Sciences Center and Attending Physician, Medical Service, James A. Haley Veterans' Hospital

merit PUBLISHING INTERNATIONAL

Cover Design and Artwork by:

SMK Design

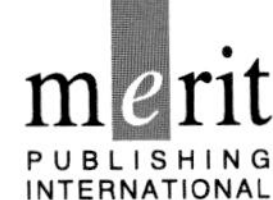

Rheumatology

Questions and Answers

MERIT PUBLISHING INTERNATIONAL

European address:
50 Highpoint, Heath Road
Weybridge, Surrey KT13 8TP
England

Tel: (44) (0) 1932 844526

Email: merituk@aol.com

North American address:
1095 Jupiter Park Drive,
Suite 7, Jupiter, FL 33458
USA

Tel: 561 697 1447

Email: meritpi@aol.com

Web: www.meritpublishing.com

ISBN: 978 1 873413 72 2

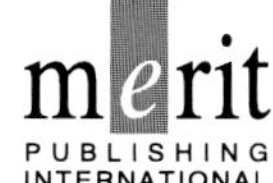

CONTENTS

Rheumatology

Questions and Answers

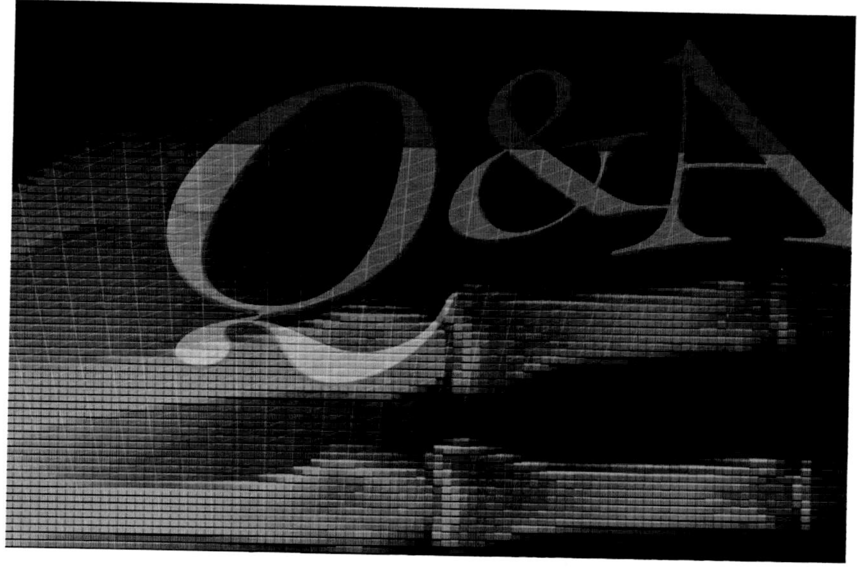

EDITOR/AUTHOR:

HAROLD M ADELMAN

AUTHORS:

JOHN D CARTER, JOANNE VALERIANO-MARCET, KEITH S KANIK, MITCHEL J SELEZNICK, BRYAN A BOGNAR, EDWARD P CUTOLO, RAJANI P SHAH

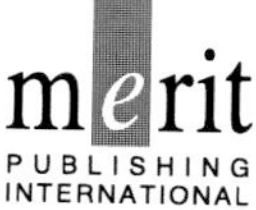

INTRODUCTION

This is an exciting time in rheumatology. The rheumatic diseases are slowly yielding their secrets to the basic sciences, and better understanding of pathogenic mechanisms is leading to more effective management of these diseases. New treatments at more fundamental biological levels are being developed. For example, in osteoarthritis, a new genre of drugs, the so-called DMOADs - disease modifying osteoarthritis drugs - is being studied. These drugs aim at promoting cartilage repair. A change in the approach to osteoarthritis is the use of acetaminophen as the first drug to choose in mild to moderate disease, for its greater GI and renal safety. In rheumatoid arthritis, several new and exciting options are now available. Various effective combinations of disease-modifying antirheumatic drugs, DMARDS, or second-line antirheumatic drugs, are being used. Potent biological agents that interfere with the *pathophysiology* of rheumatoid arthritis and other inflammatory arthritides, at a more fundamental level, have become an integral part of our armamentarium. A key change in strategy in the treatment of active, moderately severe rheumatoid arthritis is the earlier, no later than three months, implementation of this more aggressive approach to therapy.

The prognosis of systemic lupus erythematosus has improved over the past two decades. Such improvement is probably attributable to more sophisticated use of antibiotics, renal support, and intravenous pulse cyclophosphamide therapy for life-threatening disease. Maintenance hydroxychloroquine decreases major flares in lupus activity and should be used in essentially all patients with systemic lupus erythematosus unless contraindicated. Another important realization is that lupus patients are given to precocious coronary artery disease, independent of glucocorticoid use. This problem is a considerable source of morbidity and mortality in lupus patients. Consequently, aggressive coronary artery risk factor control is imperative in patients with lupus.

Proper treatment of the crystal deposition arthropathies can minimize the impact of these diseases; they are eminently manageable. The spondyloarthritides, ankylosing spondylitis being the prototype, are a group of related diseases whose immunogenetic pathogenesis is becoming better understood. Concepts such as the unfolded protein response (UPR) are being elucidated: HLA B27 is a very large macromolecule that slowly unfolds in the endoplasmic reticulum (ER). This macromolecule can get "stuck" in the ER exposing arthritogenic epitopes to immune-active cells. Better understanding of the fundamental aspects of these diseases will allow more effective treatment.

This book was written in question and answer format to stimulate learning and to enhance retention. We discuss the major entities in rheumatology and include several less common entities for their interest. It is hoped that the references will enhance presentation. The authors have pursued an international approach to epidemiology and treatment. When we refer to the American College of Rheumatology, this is an international body composed of members throughout the world. Their recommendations, therefore, apply in worldwide situations. We trust readers will find this book useful for a better understanding of the rheumatic diseases and that it will provoke new thought and research in this field.

CHAPTER 1

OSTEOARTHRITIS - DEGENERATIVE JOINT DISEASE

Harold M Adelman

Osteoarthritis (OA) is the most commonly diagnosed chronic disease in the world. It affects the majority of individuals in middle age and older. More than 80% of persons over 75 years of age are symptomatic. By X-ray, OA is almost universal by age 60 years. It has a huge economic cost, to the individual and to society and it is the single greatest causative factor of days lost from work.

OA will increase further in prevalence with the growing number of aged and obese in the population. It is high on the list of The Decade of Bone and Joint, a worldwide program initiated in Geneva in 2000 and endorsed by the United Nations.

Which joints are involved in primary osteoarthritis?

The distal and proximal interphalangeal joints of the hands, resulting in Heberden's and Bouchard's nodes, respectively, (Figure 1) and the first carpometacarpal (thumb base OA), hip, knee, first metatarsophalangeal and intervertebral joints are involved. The metacarpophalangeal joints are spared in primary OA.

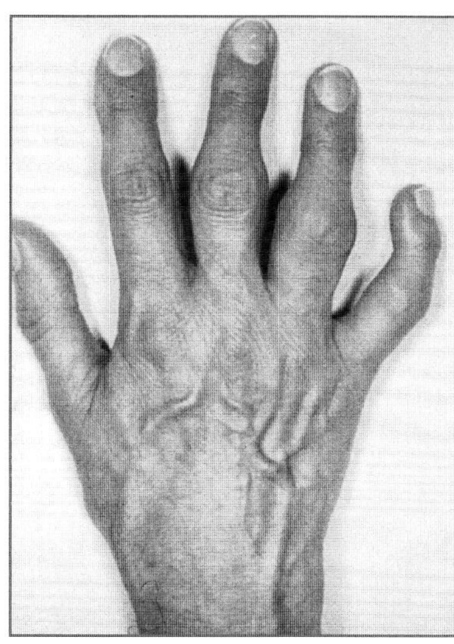

Figure 1. *Osteoarthritis. This patient's right hand demonstrates hard, bony enlargement of the third, fourth, and fifth proximal interphalangeal joints – (Bouchard's nodes.)*

If a joint other than the above is involved by osteoarthritis, which conditions causing secondary osteoarthritis should come to mind?

Prior joint damage, as by trauma or another kind of arthritis, e.g., rheumatoid arthritis, gout, pseudogout, or infectious arthritis; Paget's disease of bone; or metabolic diseases such as hemochromatosis (osteoarthritis of the second and third metacarpophalangeal joints is very suggestive of hemochromatotic arthropathy), ochronosis, or acromegaly are also to be considered.

What is the pathophysiology of primary osteoarthritis?

Osteoarthritis is essentially a disorder of cartilage, with degradation from altered chondrocyte metabolism, a decrease in glycosaminoglycans in the ground substance of cartilage, and the production of proteolytic enzymes such as matrix metalloproteinase. Importantly, there is also microfracture of subchondral bone causing stiffness and subsequent cartilage damage.

Are there genetic influences affecting osteoarthritis?

Genetic influences predispose to osteoarthritis, such as a point mutation in the gene controlling the synthesis of type II collagen, the Col2A1 gene[(1)]. As a result of the mutation, instead of sending a signal for arginine, the mutant gene codes for cysteine. In some families with spondylodysplasia and precocious osteoarthritis, this one amino acid substitution in type II collagen destroys the integrity of joint cartilage. Furthermore, Heberden's and Bouchard's nodes are heritable.

What other factors increase the risk of OA?

Age, female sex, and joint stressors such as occupation, sports activities, previous joint trauma, muscle weakness, and proprioceptive deficits, as well as genetic predisposition are risk factors for osteoarthritis.

In diagnosing osteoarthritis, what information in the patient's history and physical examination is of key importance?

The pattern of joint involvement, as discussed in the first question, is of primary importance in the differential diagnosis of joint disease: pattern recognition or pattern analysis. Heberden's and Bouchard's nodes are bony hard, whereas the joint enlargement from synovial swelling or hypertrophy of the more inflammatory arthropathies has a spongy, boggy consistency to palpation.

In contrast, in rheumatoid arthritis, the most common autoimmune arthropathy, what is the pattern of joint involvement?

In rheumatoid arthritis, the proximal interphalangeal, metacarpophalangeal, wrist, elbow, shoulder, hip, knee, ankle, metatarsophalangeal, and cervical spine joints are involved. The distal interphalangeal joints are spared in rheumatoid arthritis (Figure 2).

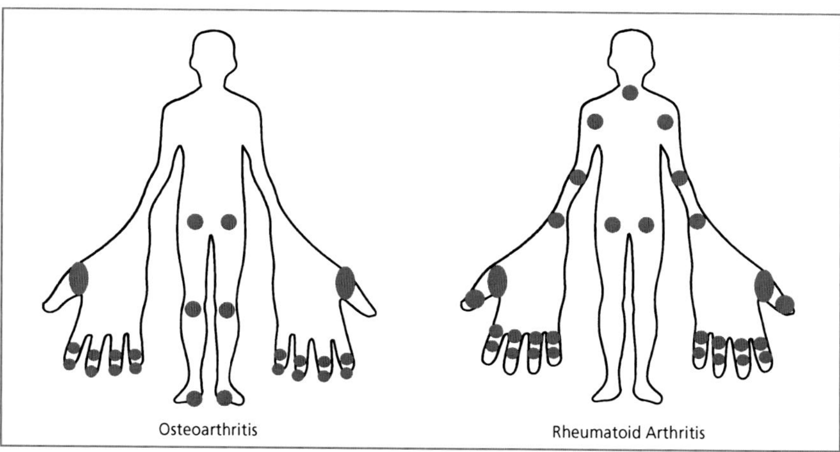

Figure 2. *This figure depicts the pattern of joint involvement in osteoarthritis (illustration on the left) and rheumatoid arthritis (illustration on the right). This pattern of involvement is central in the differential diagnosis.*

What other features of the patient's history are important in the differential diagnosis of arthritis?

In addition to the pattern or location of joint involvement, other important features of an arthropathy allowing differentiation are degree of joint pain, tempo or time to peak pain, and duration of morning stiffness. Associated signs and symptoms, e.g., constitutional symptoms such as fever, easy fatigability, poor appetite and weight loss, and the presence of rash are important distinguishing features. Likewise, kidney, nervous system, or muscle involvement with proximal muscle weakness are key distinguishing features. In osteoarthritis, the pattern of joint involvement has been discussed in question one. The tempo is insidious, usually takes years until the pain is severe. The degree of pain in osteoarthritis is usually mild to moderate until late in the course. Constitutional symptoms are usually lacking in osteoarthritis and this feature is helpful in its differentiation. For example, morning stiffness typically lasts less than 30 minutes in OA, but more than an hour in active rheumatoid arthritis.

Other examples of differentiating features are, in gout or septic arthritis, the pattern of involvement is usually one joint, especially early on in gout. The tempo is acute, with pain reaching its peak in a day or two, and the degree of pain is quite severe. Constitutional symptoms, such as fever, are common, and laboratory findings, such as an elevated peripheral white blood cell count, erythrosedimentation rate or C-reactive protein indicate a greater inflammatory process than is present in OA. Serum uric acid is usually elevated in gout. Arthrocentesis yields inflammatory synovial fluid, with the white cell count averaging 15,000 to 20,000 per mm^3 in gout and above 50,000 per mm^3 with >90% polymorphonuclear neutrophils in septic arthritis.

What do the laboratory and X-ray studies tell us in OA?

The clinical laboratory and radiology are valuable adjuncts in the differential diagnosis of OA. Laboratory tests are appropriate for the patient's age, including the CBC, erythrosedimentation rate, C-reactive protein, rheumatoid factor, and antinuclear antibody tests. Synovianalysis reveals a clear,

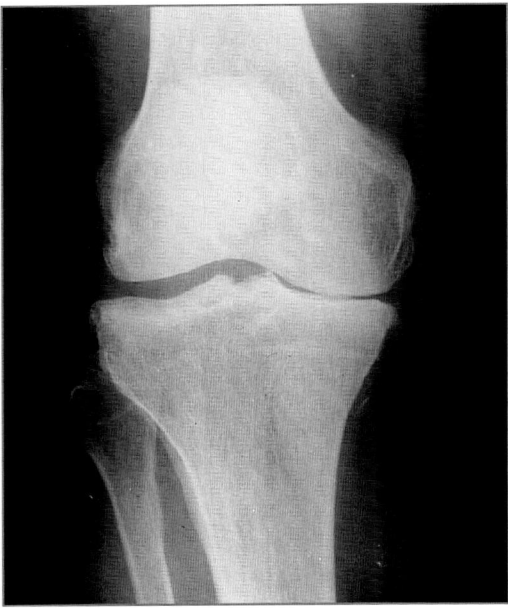

Figure 3. *X-rays of an osteoarthritic right knee. There is marked narrowing of the medial joint compartment; the lateral compartment is not narrowed.*

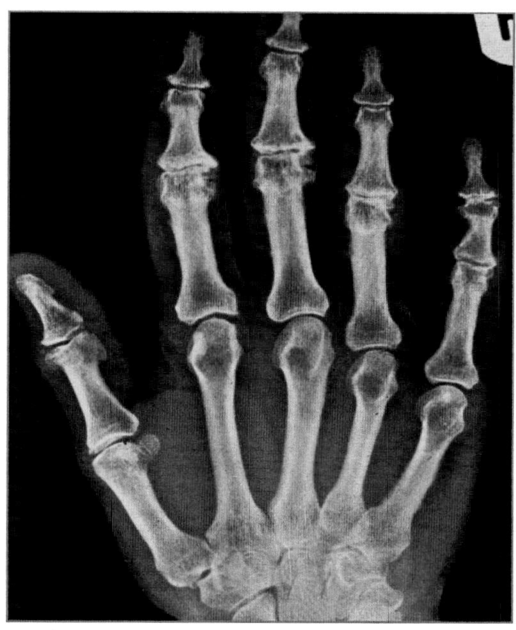

Figure 4. X-rays of a hand with osteoarthritic changes. Note joint space narrowing, subchondral bone sclerosis, and osteophyte (spur) formation.

noninflammatory joint fluid, usually with less than 3,000 white cells per mm^3. Radiology in OA typically reveals joint space narrowing, unevenly distributed in the knee (Figure 3). In rheumatoid arthritis, all three joint compartments of the knee are narrowed, the medial, lateral and patello-femoral compartments.

X-rays of the hand joints in osteoarthritis reveal sclerosis of juxta-articular bone, and there are marginal osteophytes (Figure 4). In contrast, in rheumatoid arthritis, radiology does reveal joint space narrowing, but juxta-articular demineralization instead of sclerosis, and no osteophytes (Figure 5).

If a patient with known osteoarthritis of the knee has a sudden flare of pain attended by inflammation, what concomitant of osteoarthritis should be suspected?

Calcium pyrophosphate dihydrate crystal deposition disease (pseudogout), best diagnosed by arthrocentesis and polaroscopy of the synovial fluid, is commonly the cause of an acute flare of inflammation of an osteoarthritic joint. However, other causes of acute monoarthritis, such as monosodium urate crystal deposition arthritis (gout) and infectious arthritis, also must be considered and ruled out by arthrocentesis, Gram's stain and culture of the synovial fluid, and polaroscopy.

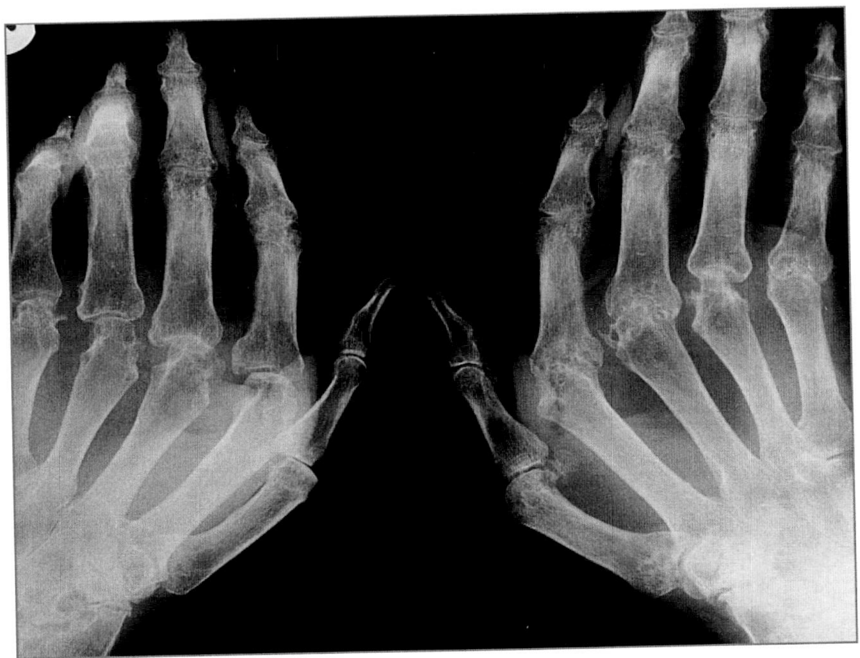

Figure 5. An X-ray of the hands of this patient with rheumatoid arthritis shows joint space narrowing and juxta-articular demineralization. There is characteristic ulnar deviation of the fingers .

What is erosive or inflammatory osteoarthritis?

An aggressive variant of OA, erosive or inflammatory OA affects the distal and proximal interphalangeal joints of the hands[2]. Blood tests are consistent with inflammation, and joint erosions appear on X-rays. Treatment requires NSAIDs, hydroxychloroquine, or prednisone[3].

What is the Milwaukee shoulder/knee syndrome?

Robert Adams in Dublin first described this arthropathy in 1857 and called it rheumatic arthritis of the shoulder. Daniel McCarty's group at the Medical College of Wisconsin in Milwaukee later named it the Milwaukee Shoulder/Knee syndrome. It typically affects older women and consists of severe osteoarthritis of one or both shoulders associated with rotator cuff degeneration, and hydroxyapatite crystal deposition. Calcium pyrophosphate dihydrate crystals might be present. Shoulder joint fluid is often blood-tinged; the fluid white cell count is low, usually <1000 per mm^3. On X-ray, there is joint space narrowing, deformity of the humeral head, small osteophytes, and indication of a rotator cuff tear (Figure 6). The knee might also be affected by destructive osteoarthritis.

Milwaukee shoulder/knee syndrome responds poorly to nonsteroidal antiinflammatory drugs or intraarticular corticosteroid injection. Joint replacement is required for severe cases [4].

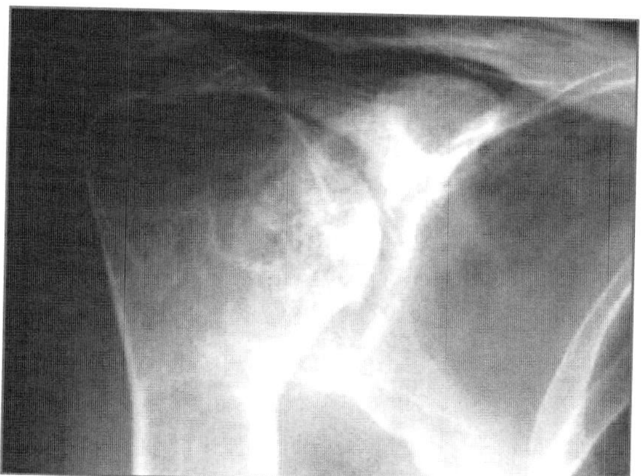

Figure 6. An AP X-ray of Milwaukee shoulder depicting the following saliencies: osteoarthritic changes, with joint space narrowing and juxtaarticular sclerosis, joint erosions, and a decrease in the acromial-humeral distance of less then 7 mm from a rotator cuff tear. Another term for Milwaukee shoulder is cuff-tear arthropathy. Deposition of calcium hydroxyapatite crystals and calcium pyrophosphate dihydrate crystals causes joint disruption.

(We gratefully acknowledge Medcyclopaedia for permision to use this radiograph.)

Two interesting endemic forms of precocious osteoarthritis are Kashin-Beck disease and Mseleni disease. What are these arthropathies?

Kashin-Beck disease is the most common arthropathy in childhood in certain parts of the world, such as Tibet, Russia, and Manchuria [5]. It is a precocious, generalized form of osteoarthritis. A high iron content in drinking water, or selenium or iodine deficiency, might play a role in its pathogenesis.

Mseleni joint disease is another precocious, progressive, generalized form of osteoarthritis starting in childhood [6]. Adults often require total hip arthroplasty. This arthropathy is endemic to the Mseleni region of Zululand, but the pathogenesis is not clear. The COL2A1 gene, and/or an abundance of type VI collagen in cartilage, might be involved.

What is the current recommended treatment of OA?

The paradigm of medical treatment of OA has changed to a more conservative approach in the last few years. Initially, in mild to moderate cases, a nonpharmacologic regimen ought to be tried, consisting of patient and family education, a judicious blend of rest and exercise, joint protection, and the use of heat or cold. Physical and occupational therapy, including splints or other orthotics as necessary, are very important where indicated. Walking and quadriceps femora muscle strengthening exercises are valuable for OA of the knee, except perhaps for people with joint laxity, or genu varus or valgus malalignments. This new concept is being elucidated at this time [7]. Weight loss for overweight patients, and general cardiovascular conditioning is of great importance for patients with OA. Wearing adhesive tape recently has been shown to reduce knee pain in OA [8]. If further treatment is necessary, acetaminophen is the drug of first choice for mild to moderate OA, in a regular dose of 4 grams daily - three 325mg tablets or two 500mg tablets qid - if there is no history of liver disease, alcoholism or malnourishment [9, 10] - conditions of decreased glutathione stores. Glutathione detoxifies the acetaminophen intermediate, N-acetyl-p-benzoquinoneimine (NAPQI). NAPQI binds to hepatocyte macromolecules, causing oxidative injury and necrosis.

Adjunct therapy might include capsaicin cream. The patient should know capsaicin takes about two to three weeks to work fully and has to be applied three or four times daily. A burning sensation is to be expected, which abates with time, and the patient warned not to allow the cream to come in contact with the eyes or other sensitive areas. These facts have to be explained to the patient so that he or she will use it correctly. It must be borne in mind that most patients with symptomatic OA are elderly and are susceptible to medication toxicity. Non-acetylated salicylates or nonsteroidal anti-inflammatory drugs in analgesic doses, which are lower than anti-inflammatory doses, are often useful and better tolerated than antiinflammatory doses of NSAIDs. Intraarticular injection of a hyaluronate or glucocorticoid can relieve a painful osteoarthritic knee. In a recent study, injecting a glucocorticoid into weight-bearing, osteoarthritic joints four times a year for up to two years did not accelerate cartilage damage [11].

Glucosamine sulfate and chondroitin sulfate look promising. In recalcitrant cases, judicious use of a narcotic analgesic and consultation with a rheumatologist and/or orthopedist are warranted. Adding tramadol with or without acetaminophen to ongoing NSAID therapy for patients with osteoarthritis can improve symptoms [12]. Furthermore, arthroplasty has given many patients with severe OA a second lease on life. An improved method of assessing patient response to treatment in OA, the patient acceptable symptom state, or PASS, measures clinically significant changes to treatment [13, 14].

What is the prognosis for patients with OA?

The notion of OA as the "noncrippling arthritis" and rheumatoid arthritis as the "crippling arthritis" is an oversimplification since both can have a mild or severe course. However, most patients with OA can lead a comfortable and productive life with appropriate management.

What is on the horizon for OA?

Disease Modifying Osteoarthritis Drugs (DMOADS) are presently being studied. This class of drugs exerts a salutary effect on cartilage, retarding joint deterioration or actually inducing a reparative response. Examples are glucosamine and chondroitin sulfate, tetracycline derivatives, risedronate, diacerin, and intraarticular injections of hyaluronan [15]. Doxycycline inhibits matrix metalloproteinase, a destructive enzyme that plays an important role in OA [16]. Gene therapy of OA is in its incipience.

STICKLER SYNDROME

What is the Stickler syndrome?

This multifaceted syndrome, also known as progressive arthroophthalmopathy, is comprised of joint pain, hyper and hypomobility of joints, joint dislocations, epiphyseal dysplasia, and precocious osteoarthritis. The ophthalmopathic component includes progressive myopia, vitreal degeneration, and retinal detachment. Other features of Stickler syndrome are progressive sensorineural hearing loss, cleft palate, and mandibular hypoplasia.

Why should we be aware of Stickler syndrome?

This autosomal dominant syndrome is not uncommon, with a prevalence of one per 10,000 in the population. It is quite under-diagnosed because many patients have a forme fruste, and a detailed family history is not always obtained.

When should we suspect this syndrome?

Stickler syndrome should be considered when there is osteoarthritis of the hip in early adulthood, or a marfanoid habitus with ophthalmopathic features, e.g. retinal detachment, with or without sensorineural deafness. A history of congenitally enlarged wrists, knees or ankles associated with a hypoplastic mandible, cleft palate, and protrusion of the tongue should bring this syndrome to mind. These last three features are known as the Robin anomalad.

What is the collagen abnormality of Stickler syndrome?

Several mutations in the type II collagen gene are recognized. For instance, the alpha1(II) procollagen locus (COL2A1) on chromosome 12 is one such site. Of interest, Stickler syndrome was the first human disease linked to a heritable defect in the collagenous component of cartilage.

KEY POINTS

- Osteoarthritis (OA) is the most common joint disease. It can be primary or secondary to other joint diseases.
- The characteristic pattern of joint involvement helps to differentiate primary osteoarthritis.
- The spine, first carpometacarpal, proximal interphalangeal, distal interphalangeal, hip, knee, and first metatarsophalangeal joints are involved in primary osteoarthritis.
- There is relatively little inflammation in most cases of OA. Consequently, there is little or no constitutional reaction, such as fatigue or anorexia.
- Laboratory tests are appropriate for the age of the patient in OA.
- Treatment is evolving. Acetaminophen has become the drug of first choice for mild to moderately symptomatic OA because of its greater GI, renal, and platelet safety profile.
- Nonsteroidal antiinflammatory drugs, weight loss, judicious exercise including water therapy, and physical and occupational therapy play a role in the optimal management of OA, as do rheumatology, physiatry and orthopedic referrals for recalcitrant cases.

CHAPTER 2

OSTEOPOROSIS

Joanne Valeriano-Marcet

What is the Socioeconomic Impact of Osteoporosis?

Osteoporosis is a systemic skeletal disorder characterized by decreased bone mass and micro-architectural deterioration of bone tissue, with a consequent increase in fragility and susceptibility to fracture (Fig 1). In the United States, one half of women and one quarter of men age 50 and over will suffer an osteoporotic related fracture within their lifetime [1]. Eight million women and 2 million men have osteoporosis with an additional 34 million Americans having low bone mass [2]. Osteoporotic fracture accounts for $14 billion in direct medical costs, > 400,000 hospital admissions, > 180,000 nursing home admissions, and two and one half million physician visits [3, 4]. In the UK, the estimated annual cost to British Health Services is one and one half billion pounds. One in three women and one in five men living to 80 years of age suffer a hip fracture from osteoporosis. There are approximately 60,000 hip fractures and 40,000 symptomatic vertebral fractures a year in the UK, mostly in Caucasians and Asians.

Vertebral fractures cause chronic pain, kyphosis, and functional limitation. They are hard to quantify as only one third come to clinical attention. Up to one half

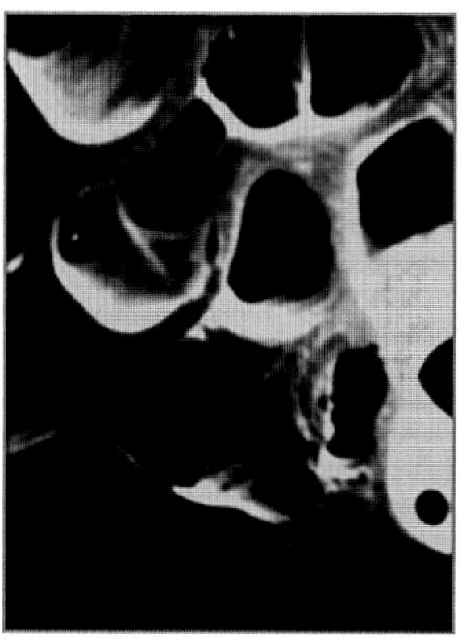

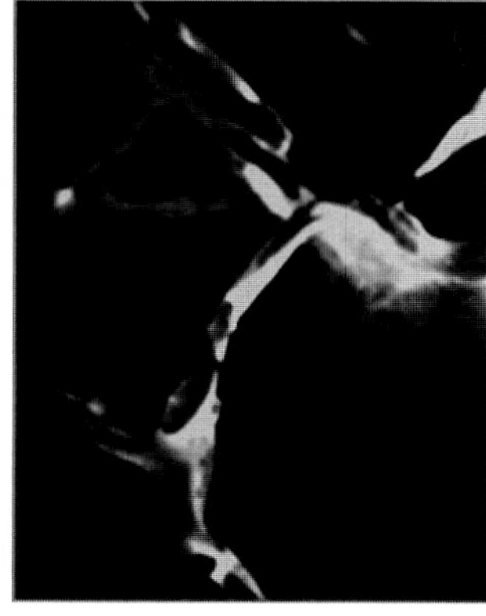

Figure 1. *Microradiograph reveals normal trabecular bone on the left and osteoporotic bone with microperforation of the trabeculae on the right.*

of patients with prior vertebral fracture experience an additional vertebral fracture within three years, many within one year. There is up to 20% excess mortality following vertebral fracture [5]. The projected annual direct cost of osteoporosis by 2040 is $50 billion [4]. Hip fracture is the most serious consequence of osteoporosis. Less than one half of hospitalized patients with hip fracture return to their pre-fracture activity level.

Six months after hip fracture only 15 % of patients can walk unaided. There is a 10-24% excess death rate the first year following hip fracture. Mortality in men is 31% compared with 17 % in women [6].

What are the Clinical and Radiographic features of Osteoporosis?

Table one summarizes the clinical features of osteoporosis.

Table 1. Osteoporosis – Clinical Features

- Asymptomatic
  Deceased bone mineralization, with or without fracture
- Compression vertebral fractures with height loss
- Thoracic and lumbar pain from fractures
- Femoral neck fracture
- Distal radius fracture
- Sacral pain from insufficiency fracture

Vertebral fractures cause sudden, severe pain localized to the site of fracture. The acute pain resolves within a few weeks, however, chronic pain may persist for years even in the absence of new fractures.

Progressive anterior vertebral compression deformity results in an exaggerated dorsal kyphosis and a characteristic deformity called a" dowagers hump". Many patients lose height from asymptomatic vertebral fractures. Figure 2 illustrates the structural changes that occur with vertebral osteoporosis. There is increased thoracic kyphosis, loss of shoulder elevation due to altered starting angle of the scapula, forward flexion of the neck, approximation of the rib cage to the pelvis, and a change in the center of gravity. These skeletal changes lead to restrictive lung disease, and a protuberant abdomen with early satiety, bloating and nausea. Hip fractures account for most of the morbidity, mortality and costs associated with osteoporosis. Distal radius fractures (Colles' fracture) may be

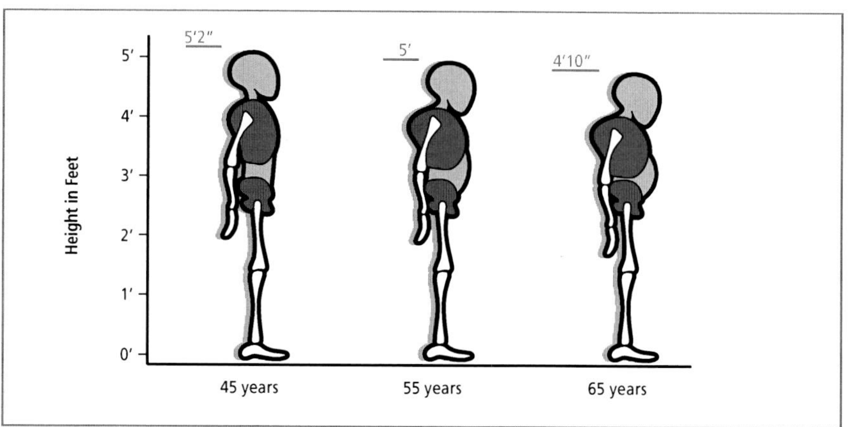

Figure 2. *Progressive loss of height from increasing osteoporotic dorsal kyphosis, the so-called dowager's hump.*

one of the first warning signs of early postmenopausal osteoporosis. Sacral insufficiency fractures present in the elderly postmenopausal women with low back and/ or pelvic pain. Plain radiographs are often nondiagnostic, and in this situation bone scanning is necessary to confirm the diagnosis.

Demineralization on plain radiographs is an insensitive indicator in early osteoporosis. Variations in technique may cause the bones to appear either denser or more osteopenic. Vertebral bodies in advanced osteoporosis lose the normal horizontal trabeculae, subsequently enhancing the vertical striations (corduroy vertebrae), Fracture of the vertebral body usually involves the anterior portion, producing flattening or wedging of the vertebrae. Osteoporotic changes seen radiographically in the proximal femur include loss of striations and a decrease in cortical thickness.

What are the risk factors for Osteoporosis?

Most risk factors for osteoporosis can fall into the categories of the physical characteristics of bone, age, heredity, gender, ethnicity, environment, endogenous hormones, and chronic diseases.

PHYSICAL CHARACTERISTICS OF BONE

Bone mass is used to define osteoporosis, subsequent bone fragility, and fracture risk. Bone strength rises as approximately the square of structural density. A 30% reduction in bone mass, as is common in osteoporosis will decrease bone strength by about 50%. Other important bone qualities include microarchitecture, composition, size, and geometry. In the case of hip fracture several aspects of gross femoral structure, such as hip axis length, cortical thickness, trochanteric width, and trabecular structure influence hip fracture risk independently of bone mass [7,14]. Several studies suggest that bone turnover as assessed by biochemical markers may be an independent predictor of fracture risk [15]. In a prospective cohort of elderly French women (≥75), urinary C-telopeptide of collagen crosslinks (CTX), and free deoxypyridinolines (Dpd) excretion above the upper limit of the premenopausal range, were associated with an increased risk of hip fracture, even after adjusting for femoral neck BMD[15].

The mechanisms by which increased bone turnover contributes to increased fracture risk include acceleration of bone loss, microarchitectural deterioration caused by perforation of trabeculae and loss of the structural elements of bone, and a reduction in bone strength caused by a larger remodeling space [16].

AGE

Bone loss is continuous throughout the aging process in both sexes. Osteoporotic fractures increase with age; wrist fractures show a rising incidence in the 50's, vertebral fractures in the 60's, and hip fractures in the 70's. Each decade is associated with a 1.4-1.8 fold increased risk of fracture. For a given bone mineral density fracture incidence increases exponentially with increasing age.

HEREDITY

The tendency for osteoporosis is hereditable. Twin studies have demonstrated this tendency, and women with a maternal history of hip fracture have a two-fold increased risk of osteoporotic hip fracture

GENDER

There is at least a two fold higher incidence among women compared with men for all age-related osteoporotic fracture sites, and men typically sustain osteoporotic fractures later in life [16-18]. Menopause with loss of estrogen is one of the major factors accounting for the higher risk of osteoporosis in women.

ETHNICITY

Ethnic variations exist in the development of osteoporosis. Black individuals have some protection against osteoporosis compared to Caucasian and Asian women[19]. Hip fracture rates are higher in white populations regardless of geographic location[16]. Hip fracture rates are lower among blacks in the United States and South Africa, and also among Japanese both in Japan and in the United States[20].

ENVIRONMENT

Nutrition: Inadequate calcium intake is believed to be an important risk factor[16]. Calcium deficiency coupled with vitamin D deficiency results in excessive parathormone secretion, which stimulates bone resorption.

Exercise: The most demonstrable interaction between physical activity and bone mass is the substantial loss that occurs with immobilization. Completely immobilized patients can lose 40% of their original bone mass in one year[21]. Trained athletes have higher bone mass than non-athletes[22]. It is important to determine whether the beneficial effects of exercise on the skeleton in athletes also occur in non-athletes. Evidence suggests that regular activity in children, adolescents, and young women positively influences bone mass[23-25]. Results of exercise studies of older people have been variable. In this population, gain in bone mineral density (BMD) in both men and women using mixed endurance/resistance training have been reported. Other studies indicate that exercise may decrease the rate of bone loss[26-28]. One of the most important benefits of exercise in the elderly is conditioning, which increases muscle strength and helps prevent falls and fractures[29].

SMOKING AND ALCOHOL

Smoking most probably affects bone mass by altering bone remodeling, and ovarian function. Alcohol is known to reduce bone mass, especially in areas of metabolically active trabecular bone[30].

MEDICATIONS

Various medications may cause osteoporosis including corticosteroids, anticonvulsants, aluminum-containing antacids, and heparin.

ENDOGENOUS HORMONES

The loss of estrogen, such as occurs with the menopause, is associated with accelerated bone loss (Figure 4). The most rapid loss occurs from two years before the last menses to three years after. The vertebral bone loss is approximately 10.5%, while total body bone loss averages 7.7%. Fifty percent of bone loss occurs a little over half a year from the last period. A similar accelerated bone loss due to gonadal hormone loss can occur in anorexia nervosa, female athletes with amenorrhea, and hypogonadal men. The over-production of corticosteroids in Cushing's Disease and Syndrome causes osteoporosis.

CHRONIC DISEASES

Chronic disease affecting the liver, kidney, and gastrointestinal tract can lead to osteoporosis. Rheumatoid arthritis is associated with decreased bone mass and increased fracture risk [31-34].

How do we use BMD testing in the diagnosis of osteoporosis? What are T scores and Z scores, and how do BMD determinations correlate with fracture risk?

Bone mineral density measurements in clinical practice reflect the amount of calcium present in the skeletal area evaluated. These values are compared with values from a reference normal population. BMD measurements do not predict fracture probability in each individual, but estimate a relative risk of fracture compared with a normal control group.

The dual energy X-ray absorptiometry (DEXA) BMD report provides the clinician with a measure of bone mineral content in grams per centimeter squared, a calculated Z score, a calculated T score, and a radiograph-like image of the site scanned. Ideally at least two skeletal sites should be tested to insure that in the individual patient a significant discordance does not exist between skeletal sites. When using the DEXA scanner, most commonly the spine and hip are selected. Many conditions may elevate the bone density reading of the lumbar spine, distorting the test readings. The most common confounders are degenerative arthritis, aortic calcifications, or artifacts such as undigested calcium tablets in the digestive tract, zippers, suspenders, clips, coins, or wallets.

A "T score" or "young adult score" refers to a comparison of the BMD of the patient being tested with a reference population of gender matched, normal young adults, and age 30-35 years. The normal T score is 0, and a T score of -1 is one standard deviation below the normal. Each standard deviation above or below normal equates to approximately 10-12 % difference in BMD. The relevance of these scores is that by definition both the National Osteoporosis Foundation (NOF) and the World Health Organization (WHO) have established criteria for the diagnosis of osteoporosis based on these scores. The science behind this information is that statistically for each standard deviation below normal BMD, the fracture risk increases by 1.9 (spine), 2.4 times (hip), and 2.7 times (forearm) [34]. The NOF defines a T score of more than 2 standard deviations below normal as osteoporosis, and a T score between 1 and 2 standard deviations below normal as "osteopenia". The WHO defines osteopenia as a bone mineral density T score between 1 and 2.5 standard deviations below normal. Although other methods besides DEXA are available for assessing bone mineral density, the T score concept applies to all currently approved technologies.

In addition to the T score, it is customary for an age- and sex- matched reference score, the Z score, to be reported. The Z score compares the patient being studied to other subjects of the same age and sex, rather than to young normal individuals as the T score does. The Z score is not being used to diagnose osteoporosis, but can be useful in following certain other conditions that affect bone mass, such as hyperparathyroidism and osteomalacia.

What other techniques are available to measure bone mineral density, and what are their advantages and disadvantages?

There are various techniques available to assess bone mineral density. The dual energy absorptiometry (DEXA) scan uses two X-ray beams, a high energy and a low energy beam. After subtraction of soft tissue absorption, the absorption of each beam is viewed and bone mineral density calculated. The technique is most widely used because of its reproducibility, accuracy, its low radiation dose, and its capacity of measuring both axial and peripheral sites [35].

Quantitative computer tomography (QCT) can provide a volumetric BMD measurement that may be more accurate, but has the disadvantages of higher radiation exposure and greater expense. Currently, only the central bone mineral density machines, DEXA and QCT, are approved for following patients serially. Peripheral bone density techniques including the ultrasound heel scanner, radiographic absorptiometry of the phalanx, and single energy absorptiometry of the forearm are approved by the FDA to screen patients for osteoporosis, These units are generally portable, easier to use and less expensive than the larger central DEXA machines. They are not used to follow repeated measurements over time, however, because of their lower precision. The precision of a test is how well that test result correlates with repeat tests results on the same sample done with the same instrument. The accuracy of a test is how well that test result corresponds to "reality" per the gold standard test.

How do we prevent and treat osteoporosis?

The phenomenon of bone loss that occurs in osteoporosis is associated with disruption of the microarchitecture and loss of trabecular elements, a process that is almost irreversible. Consequently the most effective means of intervening would be primary prevention, correcting the reversible risk factors. General measures for the prevention and treatment of osteoporosis include adequate calcium and vitamin D intake, avoidance of risk factors, and weight bearing exercise. Risk factor assessment can be used to sensitize the patient and physician to the likelihood of osteoporosis, and to target these individuals for further assessment and or treatment. Reversible risk factors should be identified discussed and modified (e.g. smoking, alcohol, and physical inactivity).

Calcium supplementation is inadequate in most people. The recommended daily calcium intake for various adult patients is seen in table 2.

Table 2. The recommended daily calcium intake for various adult patients

- Women younger than 65 – taking estrogen
  1000mg/day of elemental calcium
- Women younger than 65 - not taking estrogen
  1500mg/day of elemental calcium
- Men between 25 and 65
  1000mg/day of elemental calcium
- Women and men older than 65
  1500mg/day of elemental calcium

In order to achieve such intake, it is commonly necessary to take a calcium supplement in divided daily doses. Calcium carbonate is a highly absorbable form of calcium. If an individual is taking a hydrogen ion blocker, or proton pump inhibitor, the carbonate salt of calcium is not well absorbed, and calcium citrate should be used. Vitamin D, 400-800 IU daily is currently recommended for the prevention and treatment of osteoporosis. Intake of this level is easy to obtain through diet, multivitamins usually contain 400 IU vitamin D. Certain populations may benefit from supplemental vitamin D, including the elderly, institutionalized, and patients with disorders affecting vitamin D supply or metabolism. Examples are malabsorption, anti-seizure medication users, and patients with chronic hepatic or renal disease. Calcium and Vitamin D supplementation may help fracture prevention in the elderly [36]. In a study on female patients undergoing hip surgery for hip fracture 50% had 25OH Vitamin D levels ≤12 ng/ml (normal 15-65 ng/ml). [38] Some advocate that the "normal range" for 25OH Vitamin D may not be adequate, and higher levels (≥34ng/ml) may improve calcium absorption [36]. Regular physical activity, in addition to any potential beneficial effects on the skeleton, reduces falls and fractures, and benefits cardiovascular status.

What pharmacologic interventions are available for the prevention and treatment of osteoporosis?

Estrogen has been the mainstay for the prevention of postmenopausal osteoporosis. Estrogen can prevent bone loss; however, with the results of the Women's Health Initiative indicating an unfavorable global health index in women randomized to receive estrogen and progesterone verses placebo in a population of over 16,000 post menopausal women, the role of estrogen in the management of osteoporosis has become less clear. The combination of estrogen and progesterone increased the global index (risks exceeded benefits) by 15%, increased coronary heart disease events by 29%, strokes by 41%, venous thromboembolic disease by 111%, and invasive breast cancer by 26%. This combination decreased colorectal cancer by 37% and clinical vertebral and hip fractures by 34 % [37-40]. The decision whether to use hormone replacement to prevent postmenopausal osteoporosis needs to be tailored to the individual patient, weighing carefully the risks benefits and alternatives.

The selective estrogen receptor modulators (SERM) are a group of drugs, which bind estrogen receptors, and produce estrogen effects in some tissues (bone and lipids), and estrogen blocking effects in other tissues (breast and endometrium). Raloxifene is a SERM approved for the prevention and treatment of postmenopausal osteoporosis. In early postmenopausal women, raloxifene prevents bone loss [41].

In established osteoporosis, raloxifene decreases vertebral fracture by 40-47%. There is no proven effect on hip fracture [42]. Additional benefits include a reduction in total cholesterol and LDL cholesterol, and a 76 % decrease in invasive breast cancer [42]. Raloxifene does not prevent hot flashes, and it increases the risk of venous thromboembolus by threefold. Future studies are needed to assess the effect of raloxifene on cardiovascular disease and breast cancer risk in high-risk patients.

The bisphosphonates are a group of drugs, which bind to hydroxyapatite and inhibit bone resorption. They reduce the resorptive actions of mature osteoclasts by interfering with cell signaling, one mechanism is by stimulating osteoblastic generation of an inhibitor of osteoclastic resorption. Additionally the bisphosphonates may block recruitment and differentiation of osteoclast precursors. Alendronate and risedronate are bisphosphonates approved for the prevention and treatment of postmenopausal osteoporosis, and male osteoporosis. Risedronate is approved for prevention and treatment of steroid induced osteoporosis, while alendronate is approved for the treatment of steroid induced osteoporosis (43, 44). Both drugs prevent early postmenopausal bone loss (43-45). In patients with postmenopausal osteoporosis, they decrease vertebral fracture by 50%, and hip fracture by 40-50 % (45). They are available in once weekly forms. Due to their low intestinal absorption, and propensity to irritate the esophagus, they need to be taken first thing in the morning after an overnight fast, with a full glass of water. After ingestion, it is recommended that the individual remain upright, and avoid other food or medication for at least one half hour. Ibandronate is a more recently approved bisphosphonate indicated for the prevention and treatment of postmenopausal osteoporosis. The drug is available in oral daily and monthly or once every four-month dosages. The side effect profile and mode of administration are similar to the other bisphosphonates (46).

Calcitonin - Synthetic salmon calcitonin has been approved for the treatment of postmenopausal osteoporosis, beginning five years after menopause. It is available in intranasal and injectable forms. Intranasal salmon calcitonin decreases the relative risk of vertebral fractures in postmenopausal women with osteoporosis by 36% (47). The dose of intranasal calcitonin is 200 IU daily. It will occasionally cause nasal irritation or ulceration, so the patient should alternate nostrils with each dose.

Parathyroid Hormone- Parathyroid hormone binds to receptors on pre-osteoblasts and osteoblasts. It increases osteoblastic anabolic activity, and osteoclastic catabolic activity. Daily injection favors anabolic activity, while continuous infusion favors catabolic activity. Teriparatide is human parathyroid hormone (amino acids 1-34) made by a recombinant DNA technique. When administered by daily subcutaneous injections of 20 mcg, teriparatide decreases vertebral fractures in postmenopausal patients with osteoporosis by 65% Non-vertebral fractures decrease by 50%. There is evidence that teriparatide causes osteosarcoma in rats. Contraindications include Paget's disease, unexplained increase alkaline phosphates, open epiphyses, prior skeletal radiation, bone metastases, metabolic bone disease, and hypercalcemia. Treatment with teriparatide is indicated for postmenopausal women at high risk for fracture, previous fracture, or intolerance to other regimens. It is also indicated for men with hypogonadal or primary osteoporosis at high risk for fracture [48]. A bisphosphonate given concurrently with teriparatide can blunt the anabolic effect on bone, and thus the current recommendations are avoid concomitant use of these two medications. The maximum duration of teriparatide therapy is 18 to 24 months. Once teriparatide therapy is discontinued, use of a bisphosphonate can help to prevent the bone loss that would normally ensue.

KEY POINTS

- Osteoporosis is a systemic skeletal disease characterized by loss of bone mass and microarchitectural deterioration of bone tissue. This derangement leads to increased susceptibility to fractures.
- Most risk factors for osteoporosis fall into the following major categories: physical characteristics of bone, ageing, genetic predisposition, environmental, hormonal, and chronic morbidity.
- Bone mineral density (BMD) is one of the most important predictors of fracture risk, and is presently used to define osteoporosis.
- The T score, or young adult score, refers to the comparison of the patient's BMD with a reference population of gender matched, normal young adults age 30-35.
- The National Osteoporosis Foundation defines a T score of greater than two standard deviations below normal as osteoporosis and a T score of between one and two standard deviations below normal as osteopenia.
- The agents currently available for the prevention and treatment of postmenopausal osteoporosis include alendronate, raloxifene, and risedronate.
- Salmon calcitonin and teriparatide are available for the treatment of established postmenopausal osteoporosis.
- Estrogen is now used only for the prevention of postmenopausal osteoporosis.

CHAPTER 3

PAGET'S DISEASE OF BONE (OSTEITIS DEFORMANS)

Harold M Adelman

What is this Metabolic Bone Disease?

Paget's disease of bone is a disorder of osteoclasts of possible paramyxovirus etiology[1]. There is increased bone resorption and formation, with consequent thickened but weak bone that is hypervascular. As a result, there is bone deformity, pain and fracture. Most often, the bones of the skull, pelvis, spine, and the long bones of the lower extremities are involved and secondary osteoarthritis ensues.

What are some other Clinical Manifestations of this Disease?

Due to the hypervascularity of pagetic bone, vascular steal syndromes can occur, including a spinal artery steal syndrome. High output heart failure is a known complication of hypervascular bone. Fractures can be attended by excessive bleeding and nerve impingement can result from enlargement of bone. Deafness might be a consequence. Basilar impression can lead to hydrocephalus or signs of long tract impingement. Characteristic bony deformities such as bowed legs and enlargement of the forehead occur. Malignant transformation of pagetic bone happens in about 1% or fewer of cases. Severe pain in an area of longstanding pagetic involvement is a warning of malignant transformation, and imaging studies are indicated. Angioid streaking of the retina from rents in Brook's membrane sometimes is seen on funduscopic examination of the eyes.

What are the Characteristic Laboratory Findings?

Elevated blood alkaline phosphatase levels, a reflection of bone formation, and radiography are of primary diagnostic importance in Paget's disease of bone. It should be pointed out that many patients with Paget's disease of bone are asymptomatic, and diagnosis is made serendipitously when an elevated alkaline phosphatase is noted on routine laboratory testing in a patient without liver disease. Alkaline phosphatase is also a good way of following disease progress and response to therapy. Other biochemical tests helpful in following this disease are markers of bone resorption, e.g., collagen cross-links such as urinary n-telopeptides. Hypercalcemia can complicate Paget's disease of bone if the patient is immobilized.

How can Imaging Studies Help?

X-rays reveal the typical mosaic of bony lysis interspersed with bony sclerosis. A flamed-shaped lytic lesion of a long bone, called the *blade of grass lesion*, and a circumscribed area of osteoporosis of the cranium, called *osteoporosis circumscripta*, are characteristic X-ray findings of Paget's disease of bone. Radionuclide bone scanning is helpful in following the course of the disease.

How do we Treat Paget's Disease of Bone?

Treatment of Paget's disease of bone is with analgesics when necessary, and a bisphosphonate such as alendronate, pamidronate, risedronate, or tiludronate [(2)]. A bisphosphonate is indicated for patients at risk of complications, such as: skull involvement, the blade of grass bone lesion which portends fracture, and those whose alkaline phosphatase is markedly elevated, e.g., approximately 10 times the upper limit of normal. Duration of bisphosphonate therapy is two to three months, with all due precautions to avoid esophageal injury, and alkaline phosphatase values are checked during therapy and every three to six months thereafter. If alkaline phosphatase levels rise, another course of bisphosphonate therapy can be employed.

Is there Geographic/Ethnic Variation in Susceptibility to Paget's Disease of Bone?

Paget's disease of bone is more prevalent in Britain and in people of British lineage, with a prevalence of 6.2% in men and 3.9% in women over the age of 55. The prevalence increases with age, reaching 20% in men older than 85 [(3)]. In the United States, the overall prevalence of Paget' disease of bone is about 2%. It is less common in blacks and rare in Asians.

CHAPTER 4

OSTEONECROSIS (AVASCULAR OR ASEPTIC NECROSIS OF BONE)

Harold M Adelman

What Conditions Lead to Osteonecrosis?

Osteonecrosis results from interruption of blood circulation to bone. Some causative factors are trauma, glucocorticoid treatment by causing hypertrophy of medullary fat, which impinges on blood vessels, lupus erythematosus, with or without glucocorticoid therapy or antiphospholipid antibodies, Gaucher's disease, alcoholism, and sickle cell disease, especially sickle cell-C disease [1]. Some cases are idiopathic. There usually is increased intraosseous pressure. For the most part, the epiphyses of the femoral and humeral heads are involved, but the carpal and tarsal bones can be affected.

How does Osteonecrosis Manifest Clinically?

The pain of osteonecrosis usually occurs abruptly, and there is progressive loss of joint function. MRI is the best procedure for early diagnosis. There is high signal intensity on both T1 and T2 images with a curvilinear, serpiginous pattern. Per imaging, there are five stages of osteonecrosis. (Table One) [2].

Table 1.

- Stage 0 No signs or symptoms, normal X-ray, abnormal MRI.
- Stage I Pain, normal X-ray, abnormal MRI
- Stage II X-ray now shows osteosclerosis and osteopenia of the femoral or humeral head
- Stage III X-ray shows the crescent sign, an osteopenic line paralleling the femoral or humeral head, demarcating necrotic bone
- Stage IV More pronounced bone collapse with flattening of the femoral or humeral head, with or without secondary osteoarthritis.

How Do We Manage Osteonecrosis?

Treatment of osteonecrosis depends on the stage and extent of involvement. For stages 0 and I, conservative treatment involving analgesics, assistive devises to minimize weight bearing, and physical therapy to maintain muscle strength and prevent contractures. Medullary core decompression decreases intraosseous pressure and promotes blood flow. In more advanced stages of osteonecrosis, bone grafting can be helpful [3]. Arthroplasty is employed for severe disease and if possible, it is important to stop causative factors.

CHAPTER 5

FIBROMYALGIA

Rajani P Shah

What is the fibromyalgia syndrome?

The fibromyalgia syndrome (FMS) is the most common reason for chronic, widespread muscular pain [1]. Approximately eight million people have FMS in the United States, and primary care physicians should be able to recognize and treat this disorder. Fibromyalgia is a functional syndrome, with no particular laboratory or imaging findings. In fact, some clinicians question whether FMS is a distinct entity [2]. Patients complain of diffuse soft tissue pain and stiffness, worse in the morning, and marked tenderness to palpation at certain defined points – "tender points". Fibromyalgia can be debilitating. Non-restorative sleep characterizes fibromyalgia; patients awake not feeling refreshed [3]. It is important to get a good sleep history from the patient. Disturbed, non rapid eye movement sleep, stage three to four sleep, seems to be central to the pathogenesis of this disorder; alpha incursion on delta wave sleep is seen on EEG. A condition that disturbs the non rapid eye movement stage of sleep can lead to fibromyalgia, such as rheumatoid arthritis, Lyme disease and certain occupations, such as physicians.

Some authorities classify fibromyalgia as primary or secondary to another disease that disturbs sleep. Other factors playing a role in the pathophysiology of fibromyalgia are altered metabolism or function of the neurotransmitters serotonin, norepinephrine and substance P. Substance P is a potent vasopeptide involved in pain physiology. Serotonin down–regulates noxious stimuli by inhibiting the release of *substance P*. There are elevated substance P levels in the cerebrospinal fluid of patients with the fibromyalgia syndrome. Thus, the use of anti-depressive agents probably helps in part by increasing serotonin and decreasing substance P and nociception. Another neurotransmitter, norepinephrine, also may be involved in the pathogenesis. Tricyclic agents and tramadol affect norepinephrine at the receptor site.

Who is prone to fibromyalgia syndrome?

Fibromyalgia is one of the most common conditions seen by rheumatologists, with a prevalence of about 15% in the population. The prevalence of fibromyalgia in general medicine practice is about 5%. Primary fibromyalgia has a female predominance, >3:1, and the peak incidence occurs between the ages of 20-60. Interestingly, primary fibromyalgia has comparable prevalence rates across different countries.

What are the diagnostic criteria of FMS?

The American College of Rheumatology, an organization comprised of international members, states the criteria as follows:

- Symptoms – Widespread pain for at least three consecutive months. Widespread pain signifies pain on both sides of the body, and above and below the waist. Furthermore, there is axial pain, that is, pain in the cervical, thoracic or lumbar areas and anterior thorax.
- Signs – Marked tenderness in 11 of 18 discrete "tender points" on digital palpation firm enough to cause the examiner's fingernail bed to blanch (ca. 4 kg/cm) Figure 1. Both criteria must be present for a formal diagnosis of fibromyalgia, but a patient can have FMS without necessarily having 11 tender points. Control points such as the forehead or anterior thigh can be included in the examination for validation purposes.

What other symptoms are associated with FMS?

Associated symptoms are headache, irritable bowel, cognitive dysfunction, fatigue, and depression. Curiously, patients feel as if their joints are swollen, but on physical examination they are not inflamed

What are the aggravating and relieving factors of FMS?

Aggravating conditions include stress, inactivity and cold temperatures. Relieving factors are quality sleep, stress relief and hot showers.

What other diagnoses need to be considered in the differential diagnosis of FMS?

The American College of Rheumatology criteria for the fibromyalgia syndrome (see above) are approximately 85% sensitive and specific in distinguishing this

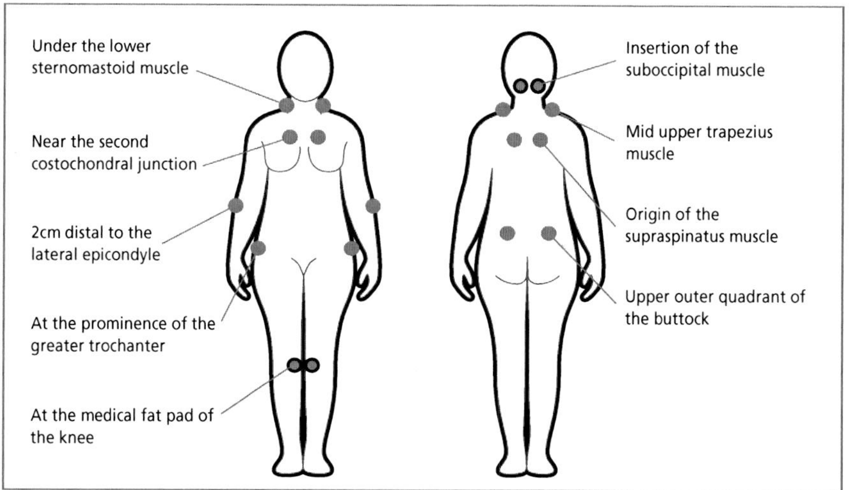

Figure 1. *The 18 tender points, 11 of which are to be present for the formal diagnosis of fibromyalgia. Exert enough pressure on the tender point so that your fingernail bed blanches.*

syndrome from other chronic musculoskeletal pain syndromes. *Hypothyroidism* can cause musculoskeletal symptoms mimicking fibromyalgia. A normal serum or plasma TSH level helps exclude hypothyroidism. *Chronic fatigue syndrome* (CFS) is an entity that must be considered when evaluating a patient with fibromyalgia. CFS is diagnosed by the chronicity, greater than six months, disabling fatigue and the exclusion of other diagnoses. The *myofascial pain syndrome* is typified by "trigger areas" (tenderness radiates from the center of the area palpated, which does not occur on palpation of a tender point) associated with a muscle twitch when the area is pressed. In this disorder, the pain is localized rather than diffuse as in fibromyalgia, and the sexes are equally affected. Other diagnoses to be entertained in the differential diagnosis of fibromyalgia are depression and anxiety, rheumatologic diseases such as polymyalgia rheumatica and early rheumatoid arthritis, and occult malignancy.

Is trauma a risk factor for fibromyalgia?

An evaluation of the literature does not support the theory that trauma per se causes fibromyalgia, with the possible exception of neck trauma.

Are silicone breast implants associated with fibromyalgia?

Current studies do not support silicone breast implants as causing fibromyalgia. Indicated in a study conducted by Wolf and Anderson in 1999, women who have had a silicone breast implant have no increased prevalence of fibromyalgia, but women with fibromyalgia are more likely to get a breast implant [4,5].

What are the current treatment strategies for the fibromyalgia syndrome?

The treatment modalities for fibromyalgia can be divided into nonpharmacologic and pharmacologic [6]. The non-pharmacologic approach includes aerobic exercises and patient and family education. This approach can be quite beneficial [7]. Assurance that FMS is not crippling or fatal is of considerable comfort to patient and family. Educational pamphlets explaining FMS are quite helpful and are available from various sources, such as the Arthritis Foundation, U.S. Arthritis Care, UK and others. Patients report improvement in pain, sleep, fatigue, and quality of life [8]. In severe cases, a multimodality approach utilizing aerobic exercise, formal cognitive behavioral therapy to alleviate harmful behavior, and consultation with a rehabilitation team, including physiatrist and physical therapist, can be very effective.

Pharmacologic therapy includes tricyclic antidepressants and cyclobenzaprine, taken one to three hours before bedtime, and/or tramadol or other narcotic analgesics used judiciously. The most commonly used tricyclic anti-depressant is amitriptyline, started at a very low dose, 5 to 10 mg one to three hours before bedtime. After two weeks, the dose is increased as necessary, by 5 mg every two weeks. Fifty mg is a dose many patients will tolerate and will find beneficial; employ the lowest dose that works. Other tricyclics used for the fibromyalgia syndrome are nortriptyline and desipramine. The mode of action is to enhance the activity of the descending pain inhibition system and to promote restorative sleep. In addition, tricyclic agents interfere with norepinephrine at its receptor. However, tachyphylaxis can occur within four months of treatment, and the medications might not work as well. Some rheumatologists use amitriptyline and cyclobenzaprine together. Fluoxetine, a selective serotonin reuptake inhibitor (SSRI), is effective as well [9]. Recently, tramadol, an opioid receptor agonist which also inhibits serotonin and norepinephrine reuptake, at a dose of 200 to 300 mg per day - with or without acetaminophen - or even opioid analgesics, have joined the armamentarium against FMS, and are being used for the control of severe, refractory pain that significantly impairs daily activities [10]. (Table one.) It is important to emphasize that these drugs must be used carefully because of side effects.

Table 1. Analgesic Progression for FMS

- Amitriptyline, cyclobenzaprine, other tricyclics
- Fluoxetine
- Tramadol with or without acetaminophen
- Oxycodone with or without acetaminophen
- Methadone

KEY POINTS

- Fibromyalgia syndrome is a very common chronic pain syndrome.
- On physical examination, eleven of eighteen tender points (see figure 1, above) are to be present to establish the *formal* diagnosis.
- Pathophysiology relates to a poor sleep pattern.
- Treatment begins with the primary care provider. It is to be emphasized to patients with fibromyalgia that most can do well with optimal treatment.
    - First line treatment includes education, encouragement and aerobic exercises.
    - Pharmacologic treatment choices include a tricyclic agent such as amitriptyline - with or without cyclobenzaprine - SSRIs (fluoxetine), tramadol with or without acetaminophen, or, as a last resort, narcotic analgesics.
    - Patients not responding satisfactorily should be referred for treatment with a multimodality approach.

CHAPTER 6

THE AMYLOIDOSES

Harold M Adelman

This chapter is dedicated to the memory of my mother, who succumbed to this disease.

What is amyloidosis?

The amyloidoses are a group of diseases characterized by the extracellular deposition in and parenchymal destruction of various organs by polymers of insoluble fibrils. So far, 21 different disease–specific protein precursors have been identified as capable of forming fibrils of insoluble, beta-pleated sheets **(a beta-pleated sheet consists of strands of polypeptides in zigzag or antiparallel formation on X-ray diffraction)**, the parenchymal deposition of which constitutes the amyloidoses[1]. The German pathologist Rudolf Virchow thought the homogenous eosinophilic material that stained with iodine was a starch, and so called it "amyloid" 150 years ago.

Which amyloidoses is the clinician most likely to see?

Amyloid L (AL) disease, formerly called primary amyloidosis, amyloid A (AA) disease, formerly called secondary amyloidosis, amyloid beta2-microglobulin disease, and the familial amyloidoses are the most commonly seen amyloidoses in clinical practice. In Alzheimer disease, the amyloid plaques are composed of amyloid beta protein, Aß.

What are the clinical manifestations of the amyloidoses?

The signs and symptoms of the amyloidoses depend on the organ, rate and amount of deposition of amyloid fibrils. The kidneys, heart, liver, skin, intestines, joints, peripheral nerves, brain, aorta, cornea, pituitary gland, and islets of Langerhans are among the organs affected by the amyloidoses.
In amyloid L disease the protein precursor is the light chain of immunoglobulin molecules, which is produced in excess. This kind of amyloidosis can be the result of either a plasma cell dyscrasia or frank multiple myeloma. Nephropathy

is a common presentation, with hypertension, nephrotic syndrome and uremia possibly eventuating. The kidneys can be small, normal or large. Cardiomyopathy is another common presentation of AL disease. Diastolic dysfunction precedes systolic dysfunction, and the echocardiogram may show a characteristic sparkling pattern. A restrictive cardiomyopathy eventuates and conduction defects and arrhythmias are common. Diagnosis is facilitated by endomyocardial biopsy with appropriate staining, see section on diagnosis below. It should be pointed out that digitalis and nifedipine toxicity is a real risk in patients with amyloid cardiomyopathy because of the penchant of amyloid fibrils to bind these medications.

Neurologic manifestations of AL disease include carpal tunnel syndrome, peripheral polyneuropathy and autonomic dysfunction including orthostatic hypotension. Arthritis from synovial amyloid deposits, resembling rheumatoid arthritis, and periarticular amyloid deposition, causing **enlarged shoulders**, the so-called shoulder pad sign, may be articular manifestations of amyloidosis. A bleeding diathesis from amyloid fibrils binding clotting factor X is a problem in some patients. The "raccoon sign," **periorbital ecchymoses** after straining, such as after a colonoscopy, is the result of blood vessel fragility from amyloid deposition. There can be malabsorption from intestinal involvement[2]. Macroglossia, an **enlarged tongue** from amyloid deposition, is characteristic of AL disease. Speech might be affected, and the tongue feels firm on palpation. The usual treatment of AL disease is with melphalan and prednisone, as for multiple myeloma, allowing prolonged survival but no cure. The course is worsening disease and death over months to years. Other treatments are currently in the pipeline.

Amyloid A disease occurs in people with chronic inflammatory conditions, with accumulation of the amyloid fibril precursor serum amyloid A, an acute phase reactant synthesized by the liver in response to elevated levels of interleukin 6. Rheumatoid arthritis, tuberculosis, osteomyelitis, and familial Mediterranean fever (FMF) are examples of chronic inflammatory diseases that can lead to AA disease. About 2% of patients with rheumatoid arthritis develop clinical renal or hepatic amyloidosis. In Sephardic Jews and Turks who develop familial Mediterranean fever, characterized by recurrent fever, joint pain, and abdominal and pleuritic pain, renal amyloidosis is a common cause of death. Colchicine has proven to be a real boon in preventing renal disease. Why amyloidosis occurs in Sephardic Jews and Turks more than in other ethnicities who develop FMF, such as Ashkenazi Jews, is not clear. Genetic differences in the mutations in the MEFV gene on chromosome 16, which encode the protein pyrin, or marenostrin, might explain this difference. The treatment of AA disease is, when possible, control of the underlying chronic inflammatory disease.

Dialysis-related amyloidosis is caused by the deposition of beta-2 microglobulin amyloid fibrils. This kind of amyloidosis is usually seen in patients on hemodialysis for at least seven years. Carpal tunnel syndrome is a usual presentation. Fractures from bone cysts of the carpal bones and the ends of long bones, such as the femoral and humeral heads, acetabulum, tibial plateau, and distal radius, caused by amyloid deposition are a major problem. These cysts are easily confused with brown tumors of the hyperparathyroid bone disease of renal failure. Curettage and bone grafts of amyloid cysts have been helpful in some cases, as has arthroplasty. Scapulohumeral periarthritis from amyloid deposition in the synovium of the shoulders can be very painful, and arthroscopic synovectomy is often helpful. The knees are affected in some patients, with a noninflammatory effusion. The cervical spine can be involved, with pain and radiculopathy. MRIs are useful in detecting cervical lesions.

A possible mechanism contributing to the bio-incompatible cuprophane dialysis membrane stimulation of ß2-microglobulin levels greater than those seen in renal disease without dialysis is activation of late complement components and cytokine formation. In a study attempting to prevent amyloid beta2-microglobulin disease, use of a polysulfone membrane dialyzer reprocessed over 24 times was associated with lower beta2-microglobulin levels [(3)]. Thus, biocompatible, noncuprophane high flux dialyzer membranes stimulate less beta-2 microglobulin synthesis and might avoid dialysis-related amyloidosis. In another study, nighttime hemodialysis for eight hours, six times a week significantly reduced plasma beta-2-microglobulin levels compared with conventional hemodialysis performed for four hours, three times a week [(4)]. The serum level of beta-2 microglobulin is not entirely responsible since not all patients with high levels develop beta-2 microglobulin amyloid disease, and the entire mechanism is to be elucidated.

Various transthyretin mutations are responsible for the many types of **familial amyloidotic polyneuropathies (FAP)**. Organs other than the peripheral nervous system are affected, such as the heart and kidney, and there can be vitreous opacities. The transthyretin mutation, methionine substitution for valine at position 30, is responsible for the majority of cases of FAP. There are unique types of FAP that occur in Sweden, Japan and Portugal[5]. **Isolated cardiac amyloidosis** in African-Americans older than 60 years of age has been described due to a variant-sequence transthyretin mutation, isoleucine for valine at position 122. The prognosis for this type of amyloidosis is varied[6]. Approximately 4% of African-Americans, 1.3 million persons, are carriers of this variant transthyretin, and are at risk for this disease.

What is the pathogenesis of the amyloidoses?

Amyloidosis is a **conformational disease**[7]. Soluble precursors undergo **conformation changes** to the insoluble polymers. **Misfolding**, leads to the characteristic **beta-pleated (antiparallel or zigzag) sheet configuration**. Fibrillogenesis is facilitated by acidification or proteolysis, and deposition of substances such as glycosaminoglycans and serum amyloid P-component.

How is amyloidosis diagnosed?

Biopsy and tissue staining with Congo red helps in the diagnosis. Good yield biopsy sites include abdominal subcutaneous fat, obtained with simple needle aspiration, rectum, bone marrow, and endomyocardium. There is a characteristic apple-green fluorescence with Congo red staining of tissue examined under polarized light. Electron microscopy demonstrates rigid, non-branching fibrils 7.5 to 10 nm in diameter. The type of amyloid fibril can be further defined by immunohistology or immunoelectron microscopy.
All amyloid deposits contain serum amyloid P (SAP) component, a glycoprotein that binds to amyloid irrespective of the protein of origin. Scintigraphy with radiolabeled SAP is a diagnostic means of detecting amyloid deposits.

Is there effective treatment for systemic amyloidosis?

At this time, treatment of the systemic amyloidoses is suboptimal. In AL disease, inhibiting excess synthesis of immunoglobulin with melphalan and prednisone slows down the course of this invariable fatal disease. In a recent study of 312 patients with AL amyloidosis at one center in North America, a regimen of high dose melphalan and autologous hematopoietic stem cell transplantation resulted in complete remissions in 40 percent but a 100 day mortality rate of 13 percent[8]. In AA disease, treatment of the underlying inflammatory disease or infection is often effective, unless the deposition of AA amyloid has progressed too far. In familial Mediterranean fever in Sephardic Jews and Turks, colchicine inhibits the acute febrile attacks and overproduction of the amyloid precursor serum amyloid A. Consequently, colchicine can prevent the fatal kidney involvement in this particular amyloidosis. Colchicine can also reverse other organ dysfunction from amyloid deposition in this disease. Unfortunately, colchicine has proven ineffective in treating other kinds of amyloidosis. In the transthyretin-associated amyloidoses, liver transplantation can be effective if performed before there is heart involvement.

What does the future hold?

As we understand the structural abnormalities and pathogenesis of the amyloidoses, research for more effective treatment appears encouraging. Inhibiting the misfolding of fibrils into the insoluble polymers by stabilizing ligands is currently being studied. "Beta-busting" is an attractive approach, that is, to rearrange the insoluble zigzag configuration of amyloid fibrils to a soluble parallel configuration. Clearing serum amyloid P component, SAP, from amyloid fibrils is currently in phase 2 clinical trials. Another approach being considered is immunization against fibrillar proteins. This process enhances the clearance of amyloid deposits.

KEY POINTS

- The amyloidoses are a group of diverse diseases that result from the deposition of insoluble fibrils in various organs.
- Amyloid L disease, also known as primary amyloidosis, results from the misfolding and accumulation of precursor immunoglobulin light chain molecules, and is seen in plasma cell dyscrasias and multiple myeloma.
- Amyloid A disease, also known as secondary amyloidosis, results form the misfolding and accumulation of the precursor acute phase reactant, serum amyloid A.
- Amyloid A disease is seen in chronic infections, such as tuberculosis and osteomyelitis, and in chronic inflammatory diseases, such as rheumatoid arthritis and familial Mediterranean fever.
- It is important for the clinician to be aware of several other kinds of amyloidosis, such as amyloid beta2-microglobulin disease seen in dialysis patients with end stage renal disease and the transthyretin mutation-driven amyloidoses, examples of which are the familial amyloid polyneuropathies and the amyloidosis causing isolated cardiac amyloidosis in African-Americans older than 60 years of age.

- Diagnosis most commonly relies on staining of biopsied tissue with Congo red. Under polarized microscopy, there is apple-green birefringence with Congo red staining.
- Current treatment of the amyloidoses is of varying effectiveness, depending on the type of amyloidosis. For AL disease, melphalan and prednisone allow prolonged survival but not a cure.
- For AA disease, treating the underlying chronic inflammatory disease or infection can be curative. Liver transplantation can be curative for the transthyretin mutation-driven amyloidoses if advanced cardiac involvement has not yet occurred.
- For the amyloidosis of familial Mediterranean fever, colchicine can be dramatically effective if advanced renal disease has not yet transpired.

SECTION TWO

INFLAMMATORY, AUTOIMMUNE RHEUMATIC CONDITIONS

CHAPTER 7

RHEUMATOID ARTHRITIS

Keith S Kanik

What is rheumatoid arthritis?

Rheumatoid arthritis is an autoimmune, inflammatory disease. It is defined by the American College of Rheumatology by the presence of at least four of the following seven criteria [(1)]:

- Morning stiffness of one hour or greater
- Arthritis of three or more peripheral joints
- Arthritis of the hand joints (Figure 1)

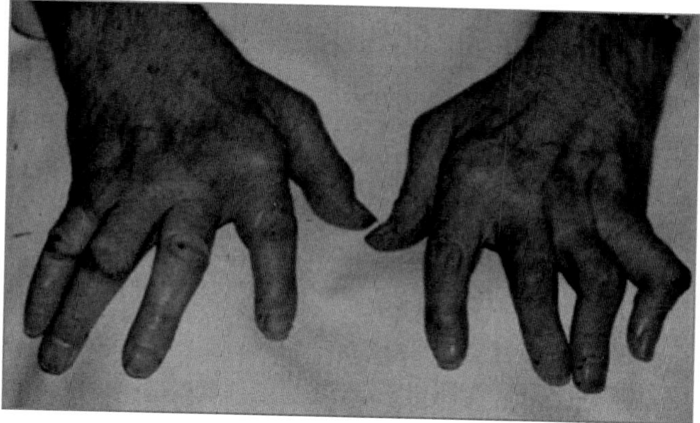

Figure 1. Early rheumatoid arthritis of the hand. A strong clue that this patient most likely has rheumatoid arthritis is the pattern of joint involvement. The proximal interphalangeal and metacarpophalangeal joints are involved, and the distal interphalangeal joints are spared. Other arthropathies can appear this way, such as that of systemic lupus erythematosus or patients with the polyarticular pattern of psoriatic arthritis. A careful history and physical examination, the cornerstone of all diagnoses, will help focus on the right diagnosis.
©1972-2004 American College of Rheumatology Clinical Slide Collection. Used with permission.

- Symmetric arthritis
- Rheumatoid nodules (Figure 2)
- Rheumatoid factor in serum
- Typical radiographic abnormalities (Figure 3, 4).

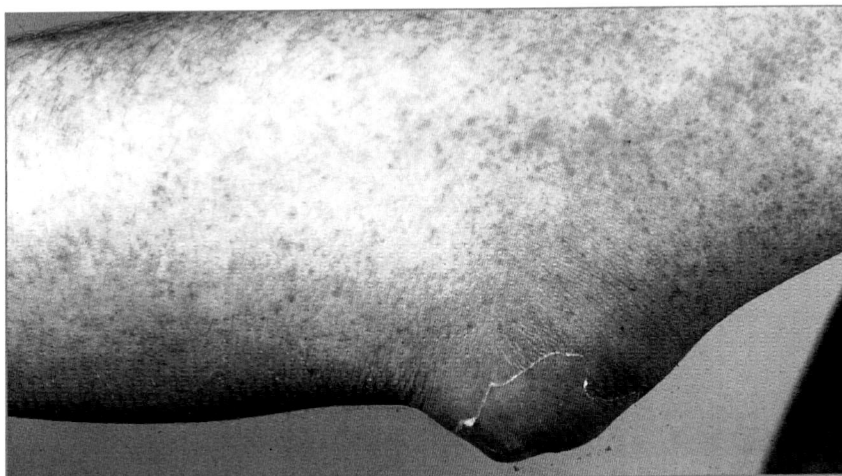

Figure 2. *The olecranon bursa is a characteristic site of a rheumatoid nodule. These nodules tend to form in areas of friction, especially over the elbow, extensor surface of the forearm, and Achilles tendon. Gouty tophi are indistinguishable on inspection.*

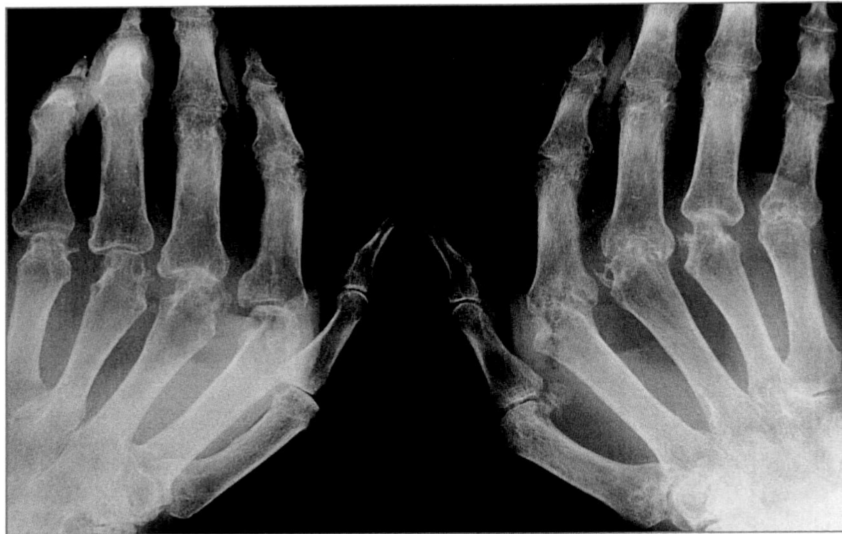

Figure 3. *This X-ray of a patient's hands shows ulnar deviation, joint space narrowing, and juxtaarticular demineralization. The wrists, metacarpophalangeal and proximal interphalangeal joints are involved. The distal interphalageal joint appear to be involved, but there is positioning artifact.*

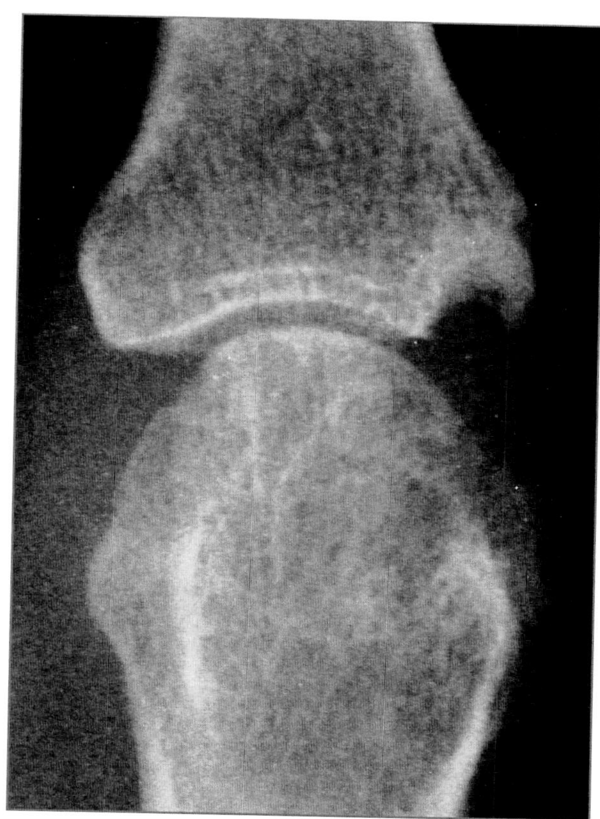

Figure 4. *A magnified view of a proximal interphalangeal joint demonstrates typical marginal joint erosion in rheumatoid arthritis.*

These criteria are useful for studies and epidemiologic data gathering, and it should be emphasized that RA can be diagnosed in the individual patient without meeting four criteria.

The synovitis of rheumatoid arthritis, and other inflammatory arthropathies, is characterized by a soft tissue swelling that is boggy or doughy in consistency, not the hard, bony hypertrophy characterizing osteoarthritis.

Again pattern recognition is of key importance in diagnosing RA (Table 1). Namely, early in the course, RA characteristically involves small joints, such as the proximal interphalangeal (PIP), metacarpophalangeal (MCP) and wrist joints. There is spindle-shaped or fusiform swelling of the PIP joints (Figure 1). The **ulnar styloid process** is a favored target in RA. There is a more or less symmetric pattern of joint involvement. Table one summarizes the joints involved in rheumatoid arthritis and some of the clinical manifestations.

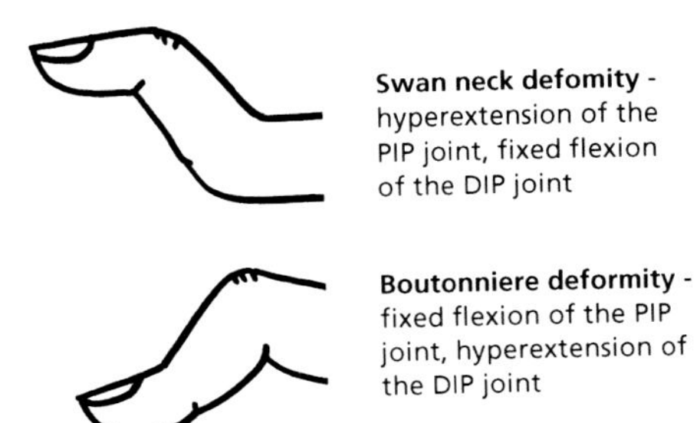

Other classic hand deformities in RA are ulnar deviation and swan neck and boutonniere deformities
Swan neck defomity - hyperextension of the PIP joint, fixed flexion of the DIP joint
Boutonniere deformity - fixed flexion of the PIP joint, hyperextension of the DIP joint

Figure 5a. The top finger demonstrates a swan neck deformity. There is flexion of the distal interphalangeal joint, as if a swan were admiring its reflection in a lake, and extension of the proximal interphalangeal joint.

Figure 5b. The bottom finger demonstrates a boutonnière deformity, in which the opposite deformities occur. There is extension of the distal interphalangeal joint, as if the finger were pushing a flower though the button hole of a dinner jacket, and flexion of the proximal interphalageal joint. Because of chronic synovitis, there is tendon slippage, and the hand deformities depend on the direction of slippage.

Table 1. Joints Involved in RA

JOINT	COMMENTS
Cervical Spine	Can cause cervical myelopathy or protrusion of the dens into the foramen magnum
Cricoarytenoid	Can cause stridor and asphyxiation
Shoulders	
Elbows	Ulnar nerve compression
Wrists	Median nerve compression with carpal tunnel syndrome. Ulnar styloid process involvement
Metacarpophalangeal	Characteristic, early involvement
Proximal Interphalangeal	Characteristic, early involvement
Hips	
Knees	Popliteal (Baker's) cysts can complicate involvement of the knees, with pseudo-thrombophlebitis if the cyst dissects down the calf
Ankles	
Feet	

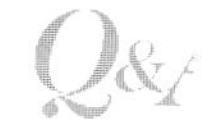

What is the prevalence of RA?

The prevalence is practically consistent worldwide at about 1%. Exceptions are a very low prevalence in much of Africa, and a high prevalence, about 5% or more, in the Yakima and Chippewa Amerindians, who have a high frequency, about 70% of HLA class II alleles associated with susceptibility to rheumatoid arthritis. In American Caucasoids, the frequency of HLA-DR4 is about 30%.

What does a positive rheumatoid factor mean?

A positive rheumatoid factor, by itself, does not make the diagnosis of RA. In conjunction with symmetric arthritis or other typical clinical signs noted above, it could help confirm a diagnosis. High titers of rheumatoid factors correlate with more aggressive joint disease, as well as extraarticular manifestations of RA, such as subcutaneous nodules, scleritis, and vasculitis[2]. About 5% of patients with RA develop AA amyloidosis, which can lead to fatal renal involvement. Serum rheumatoid factor is not a specific test, as it can be positive in other conditions of chronic immune stimulation.

What is the clinical utility of the new anti-cyclic citrullinated peptide (CCP) antibody assay?

Citrulline is derived from arginine by deamination. The anti-CCP antibody assay is a test that is more specific than rheumatoid factor for rheumatoid arthritis, 90.4% vs 80.3% but it is less sensitive, 66% vs 71.6%. If both anti-CCP and rheumatoid factor assays are used, testing sensitivity for RA increases to 81.4%, as 34% of rheumatoid factor negative rheumatoid arthritis patients are positive for anti-CCP antibodies. Anti-CCP antibodies also correlate with prognosis; patients with this autoantibody tend to have more aggressive disease. The anti-cyclic citrullinated peptide antibody test is becoming more readily available, and it will be useful in the earlier diagnosis and in gauging prognosis in RA[3].

What is the shared epitope, and how is it germane to the pathogenesis and severity of Rheumatoid Arthritis?

An epitope is a site on the surface of an antigen to which a single antibody molecule binds. Several alleles at the class II major histocompatibility complex DRB1 locus contribute to the susceptibility to rheumatoid arthritis. In particular, the combination of HLA DRB1*0401 and HLA DRB1*0404 confers a relative risk of 60 times of developing rheumatoid arthritis. The "shared epitope" connotes a similar five-amino acid sequence at positions 70 – 74 of several DRB1 alleles that is associated with RA. This five-amino acid sequence is mainly glutamine, arginine, arginine, alanine, and alanine. Lysine is at position 71 of HLA DRB1*0401. Crystallographic studies have demonstrated a structural cleft in these DRB1 molecules where it can bind and efficiently present arthritogenic peptides to T cells. Another possible explanation for the increased risk of developing RA with these alleles is that they regulate the peripheral T cell repertoire by acting to select for particular T cell receptors during thymic selection.

In rheumatoid arthritis, is there organ involvement other than the joints?

Yes and this fact is very important to recognize. Several of these manifestations are potentially life threatening and require more aggressive treatment, e.g., high doses of prednisone (1 mg/kg/day). Some authorities call rheumatoid arthritis rheumatoid disease because of the multisytem involvement. (Table 2)

Table 2. Extra-Articular Manifestations of RA

INVOLVEMENT	SELECTED MANIFESTATIONS
Skin	Rheumatoid Nodules – paradoxically, methotrexate may accelerate rheumatoid nodule formation; skin ulcers; palpable purpura
Eyes	Keratoconjunctivitis sicca (part of secondary Sjogren syndrome) Episcleritis and scleritis with scleromalacia perforans. Scleritis portends a more virulent course.
Lungs	Pleuritis +/- pleural effusion with very low glucose levels Interstitial pulmonary fibrosis Rheumatoid nodules in the lung, which may cavitate, +/- bronchopleural fistula Bronchiolitis obliterans
Heart	Pericarditis; cardiomyopathy; aortitis +/- aortic insufficiency; myocardial infarction
Gastrointestinal	Xerostomia (part of secondary Sjogren syndrome) Ischemic bowel from rheumatoid vasculitis

Table continued overleaf

INVOLVEMENT	SELECTED MANIFESTATIONS
Renal	The kidneys are usually spared in rheumatoid arthritis unless injured from treatment toxicity or from AA amyloidosis.
Neurological	Cervical spine instability, e.g., atlanto-axial subluxation from ligamentous laxity with cervical myelopathy, and protrusion of a whittled dens into the foramen magnum, which can be fatal. A mild distal sensory neuropathy Carpal tunnel syndrome
Vasculitis of the vasa nervorum	Mononeuritis multiplex with foot or wrist drop
Hematological	Anemia of chronic disease Eosinophilia, which correlates with disease severity Lymphadenopathy, which can mimic a lymphoma Lymphoma Felty syndrome, with neutropenia and splenomegaly Large granular lymphocyte syndrome
Systemic necrotizing rheumatoid vasculitis	See text
Constitutional symptoms	Fever, easy fatigability, general malaise, poor appetite, weight loss

What is Rheumatoid Vasculitis?

Rheumatoid vasculitis can involve small vessels, small muscular arteries as a localized vasculitis- an example of which is periungual infarcts, so-called Bywater's lesions that may or may not indicate a more wide-spread, systemic vasculitis; or a systemic, life threatening, necrotizing vasculitis involving medium-sized arteries similar to polyarteritis nodosa. The latter is seen more in men with high titer rheumatoid factor and subcutaneous nodules. The GI tract, heart, liver and kidney are among the target organs of systemic, necrotizing rheumatoid vasculitis.

What is Felty syndrome?

This syndrome is characterized by seropositive rheumatoid arthritis associated with neutropenia and usually splenomegaly. There are often recurrent infections, leg ulcers, and pretibial hyperpigmentation. Part of the spectrum of Felty syndrome is the *large granular lymphocyte syndrome*, which is a lymphoproliferative disorder [4] .

What is adult onset Still's Disease?

Adult onset Still's disease (AOSD) is a seronegative (rheumatoid factor negative and ANA negative) arthritis associated with high fever, sometimes with one or two daily temperature spikes - a double quotidian fever, and a **tell-tale evanescent, salmon-colored rash** that lasts minutes to hours. Still's disease in children is also known as systemic juvenile rheumatoid arthritis. The prevalence **in adults** is one per one million of the population, and it usually occurs before the age of 35 years. However, cases have been reported in individuals in their 70s. In some series, adult Still's disease comprises 15% of cases of **fever of unknown origin**, and the characteristic rash is important in making the diagnosis. The knee and wrist are the most commonly involved joints, but interestingly, the distal interphalangeal joints are involved in 20% of patients with AOSD. The diagnosis of AOSD is supported by the presence of very high serum ferritin levels, which can reach over 10,000 ng/mL - normal value ranges from 40 - 200 ng/mL, and a low fractional glycosylation of ferritin, less than 20%. In one study, the combination of a five-fold or greater elevation of serum ferritin and a glycosylated fraction less than or equal to 20% had a sensitivity for AOSD of 43% but a specificity of 93% [5]. A total ferritin level over 3000 ng/mL is not seen in other rheumatic diseases. A glycosylated ferritin assay is not performed in most labs. AOSD is a multisystem disease, with pleuritis, lymphadenopathy, hepatosplenomegaly, elevated hepatic aminotransferases, anemia, and a peripheral leukocytosis, predominantly neutrophils. The metacarpal-carpal joints can become ankylosed. Treatment is similar to that of RA, and some patients may respond to high dose salicylates alone. Anakinra seems to be effective in this disease.

There are several published sets of criteria for the diagnosis of adult onset Still's disease. Those of Yamaguchi et al are practical (Table 3). These criteria are also 90% sensitive when five criteria, three or more being major, are present. Exclude malignancy, infection and vasculitis. Whether adding hyperferritinemia to the criteria will improve specificity is not yet clear.

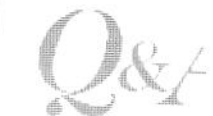

Table 3. Criteria for the Diagnosis of Adult Onset Still's Disease

MAJOR CRITERIA	MINOR CRITERIA
Temperature of >39°C for >1 wk	Sore throat
Leukocytosis >10,000/mm^3 with >80% PMNs	Lymphadenopathy
Evanescent, salmon-colored macular or maculopapular rash	Splenomegaly
Arthralgias >2 wk	Liver dysfunction (high AST/ALT) Negative ANA and RF

Abbreviations: *ALT, alanine transaminase; ANA, antinuclear antibody; AST, aspartate transaminase; PMN, polymorphonuclear leukocyte; RF, rheumatoid factor.*
From: *Yamaguchi M, Ohta A, Tsunematsu T, et al. Preliminary criteria for the classification of adult Still's disease. J Rheumatol 1992;19:424-30.*

How do I choose an optimal therapeutic regimen for a patient with rheumatoid arthritis?

Proper treatment of RA involves patient and family counseling and education, physical and occupational therapy, and a medical regimen suited to the severity of the particular patient's course. Second-line medication, also known as disease modifying antirheumatic drugs (DMARDs), is currently recommended to be started after six weeks, to exclude RA mimics, e.g. viral arthritis, and *within three months* in most cases of persistently active rheumatoid arthritis. Earlier, aggressive treatment has a markedly salutary effect on prognosis.

RA is a potentially fatal disease and has to be treated aggressively soon after onset. Corticosteroids, both intraarticular and systemic, can be used early as bridge therapy, until the DMARD is fully effective. DMARDs may take from two to eight months to achieve maximum benefit. Chronic corticosteroid use should be kept to a minimum, as its toxicity is significant.

What is nuclear factor-kappa B?

Nuclear factor-kappa B (NF-kB) is a key transcription factor that plays a pivotal role in the activation of many genes important in RA, such as TNF-alpha and IL-6. NF-kappa B is found in the cytoplasm of cells in an inactive form coupled to an inhibitory protein called IkappaBeta. Extracellular stimuli cause phosphorylation of IkappaB, permitting NF-kappaB to migrate to the cell nucleus and bind its target genes to initiate transcription. Glucocorticoids inhibit the synthesis of cytokines, and appear to act by inducing the synthesis of a protein that inactivates nuclear factor kappa B (NF-kB).

What is the role of the nonsteroidal antiinflammatory drugs?

Nonsteroidal antiinflammatory drugs are useful in diminishing symptoms, but they have not been shown to control disease progression.

When should we start second-line therapy?

Any patient with erosions, or first-line-treatment resistant, aggressive synovitis, should be treated with methotrexate and/or another DMARD. Methotrexate is the current DMARD of choice for RA, and combination therapy with methotrexate, sulfasalazine, and/or hydroxychloroquine is used early – *within three months* - in recalcitrant cases. Changing from oral to **parenteral** methotrexate at a dose of 15-20 mg/week may lead to further improvement in some patients who have not responded satisfactorily to oral doses of 20 mg/week. Parenteral dosing improves absorption of the drug. Higher parenteral doses, up to 45 mg/week, are not more effective than a 15-20 mg/week dose [6].

Relatively recent additions to the armamentarium against rheumatoid arthritis are being employed with gratifying success. Leflunomide, a pyrimidine inhibitor, by itself or in combination with methotrexate, and biological agents, such as the tumor necrosis factor alpha blockers etanercept, infliximab, adalimumab, and an interleukin – 1 blocker anakinra, have shown efficacy in not only controlling the signs and symptoms of RA, but slowing, preventing and/or possible even reversing erosive disease [7,8,9]. It is somewhat debatable when to start these newer drugs, but they should certainly be considered early – within three months if methotrexate fails or is not tolerated [10,11]. Other targets in the treatment of recalcitrant rheumatoid arthritis are T cells and B cells. CTLA4Ig (cytotoxic T-lymphocyte-associated antigen 4) is a fusion protein that inhibits T-cell activation [12], **Abatacept** was approved by the FDA in December 2005. Targeting B cells in systemic autoimmune diseases is also a current topic of much interest in rheumatology. In rheumatoid arthritis, B cells present antigen to activate T cells. The CD20 antigen is expressed on B cells, and **rituximab**, a chimeric anti-CD20 IgG1 monoclonal antibody, became available for the treatment of refractory rheumatoid arthritis in early 2006. Studies show efficacy, including a steroid spring effect, of B lymphocyte depletion in various, refractory systemic autoimmune diseases, such a refractory RA [13], SLE, primary Sjogren's syndrome, vasculitis and polymyositis [14]. Further studies will elucidate the role of rituximab in the rheumatic diseases. See the **therapeutics chapter** for more information about these medications. If improvement is not satisfactory or sustained, switching agents can improve response. Treatment should be undertaken in collaboration with a rheumatologist.

In noting improvement, changes in sequential joint X-rays, joint space narrowing and joint erosions are quantitated (e.g., the Sharp score or the Larsen score). The American College of Rheumatology (ACR) quantitates clinical improvement in rheumatoid arthritis as an ACR-20, ACR-50, and ACR-70 improvement. These measures denote a ≥20%, ≥50%, and ≥70% improvement respectively in the tender joint count and the swollen joint count, as well as a ≥20%, ≥50%, and ≥70% improvement respectively in three of the five following criteria: patient pain assessment, patient global assessment, physician global assessment, patient self-assessed disability, and the erythrosedimentation rate or C-reactive protein.

What is the role of tetracycline derivatives in RA?

Tetracycline derivatives, such as minocycline or doxycycline, decrease destructive matrix metalloproteinase activity in the joint and have an immune modulatory effect, e.g., effects on T-cell and neutrophil function. Doxycycline should be used with methotrexate for efficacy. In one study of patients with early, seropositive rheumatoid arthritis, placebo and doxycycline in a dose of 20 mg bid or 100 mg bid led to an ACR50 response of 13, 33 and 42 percent, respectively – a statistically and clinically significant difference [15]. A recent meta-analysis showed a reduction in disease activity with minocycline but not doxycycline alone [16].

Can deformities be predicted and prevented?

The presence of a high rheumatoid factor, and/or rheumatoid nodules is often associated with more aggressive disease. Also ominous is the development of erosions within the first months of the disease. The anti-cyclic citrullinated peptide antibody test, which is becoming more widely available, is predictive of more destructive RA. The presence of certain HLA subtypes, e.g., HLA-DRB1*0401, may be predictive of more destructive arthritis; however, they are not routinely used in clinical practice. Interestingly, measures indicating functional disability, such as the Modified Health Assessment Questionnaire, as well as age and comorbidity predict five-year mortality more effectively than radiographic and laboratory data [17,18]. Current evidence strongly supports **early** – by three months of active rheumatoid disease not responding to NSAIDs - aggressive DMARD or anticytokine therapy to minimize erosive arthritis and deformities, and to delay or perhaps even prevent early mortality [8, 9]. Two recent, randomized controlled trials looked at early combination therapy and were very positive [19, 20].

KEY POINTS

- Rheumatoid arthritis (RA) is the most common autoimmune-inflammatory arthritis, with a prevalence of about 1.5%.
- The clinical hallmark of RA is the pattern of joint involvement.
- There is a symmetrical, polyarticular distribution of arthritis with a predilection for the small joints of the hands, wrists and feet early in the course.
- Treatment of RA has improved recently with the addition of several, effective new modalities.
- Another recent shift in the therapeutic paradigm of RA is the earlier (after six weeks but within three months of active disease) use of DMARD therapy and combination DMARD therapy to prevent crippling joint disease and perhaps prevent premature death.
- Some authorities favor using low dose corticosteroids, prednisone or prednisolone, ≤7.5 mg a day, for RA as well, and decreasing slowly, e.g., by 1 mg a month or slower, when the DMARD medication(s) take(s) effect.
- Beware the extra-articular manifestations of rheumatoid arthritis (Table 2).
- If a patient with rheumatoid arthritis needs surgery, lateral view X-rays of the C-spine in flexion and extension are imperative, and the anesthesiologist notified if there is atlanto-axial subluxation or whittling of the dens.

CHAPTER 8

SYSTEMIC LUPUS ERYTHEMATOSUS (SLE)

Keith S Kanik

What is Systemic Lupus Erythematosus?

Systemic lupus erythematosus (SLE) is a multisystem autoimmune disease that can affect virtually any organ in the body. It is associated with certain characteristic autoantibodies. The name lupus, Latin for wolf, comes from early descriptions of the disease as facial disfigurement -- as if maimed by a wolf. Four out of eleven criteria, as established by the American College of Rheumatology (ACR), are required for the diagnosis of lupus for clinical research purposes. It should be stressed, though, that these criteria do not apply to diagnosing the individual patient. The ACR criteria include: malar rash, discoid rash, photosensitivity, oral ulcers, serositis, arthritis, renal disorder, neurological disorder, hematological disorder, antinuclear antibody (ANA), and other immunologic laboratory abnormalities. The lupus malar rash is defined as a flat or raised, reddish purple exanthem sparing the nasolabial folds (Figure 1).

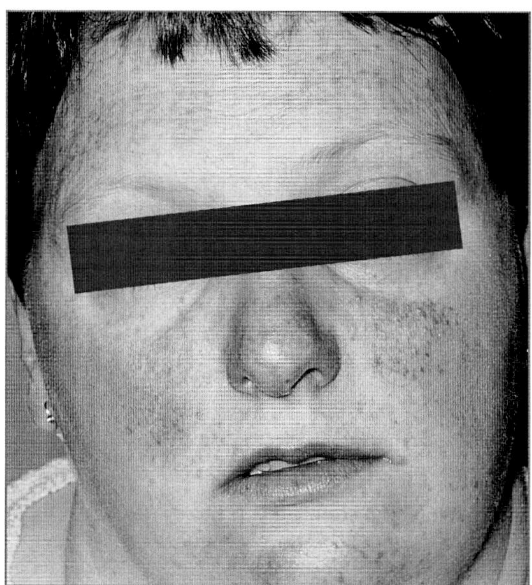

Figure 1. This woman with SLE has the characteristic butterfly rash, involving the cheeks (malar rash), bridging the nose, and typically sparing the nasolabial folds. It is not scarring. This rash can be confused with acne rosacea.

The rash of discoid lupus (Figure 2) is a reddish purple, raised, keratotic lesion that leaves a scar. It often involves the external auditory canal and scalp. Discoid lupus usually occurs in areas of the body exposed to sunlight. Photosensitivity is the development of a cutaneous exanthem (not necessarily malar or discoid) after exposure to the sun or other sources of ultraviolet light.

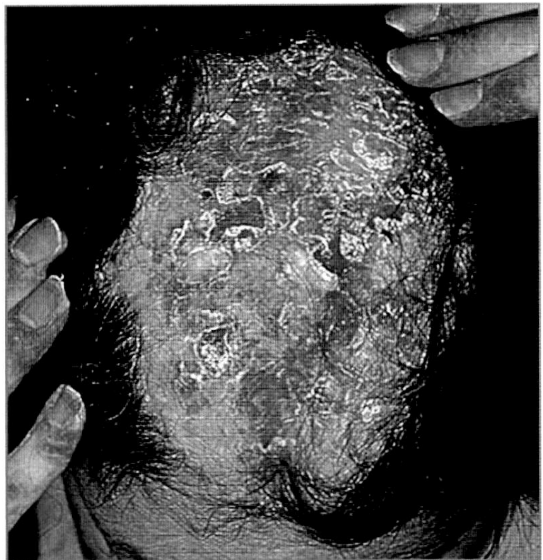

Figure 2. *This patient with discoid lupus has alopecia and a scarring rash on her scalp. There are keratotic plugs.*
Doria A, Rondinone R, University of Padova, Italy.

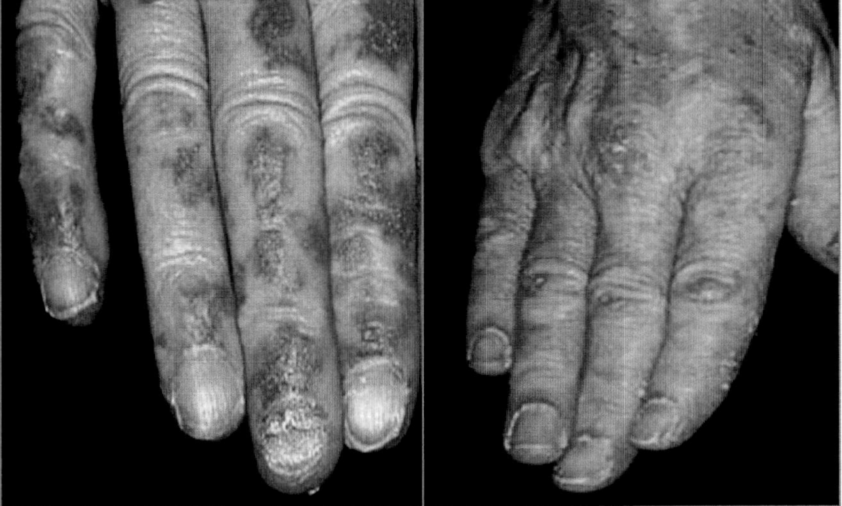

Figure 3. *Left panel - Chronic cutaneous lupus. Right panel - dermatomyositis rash of the hand.Note greater involvement of the skin between the joints in lupus, and greater involvement of the skin over the joints in dermatomyositis. Doria A, Rondinone R, University of Padova, Italy.*

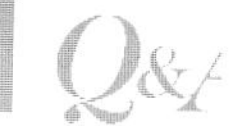

The oral ulcers of SLE are usually painless, and they are not canker sores. **Serositis** is defined as a convincing history of pericarditis or pleuritis. **Renal disorder** is defined by proteinuria greater than 0.5 grams per day or cellular casts in the urine. A recent reclassification of lupus nephritis has been published based on clinicopathologic correlations [1].

Neurological disorder includes seizures or psychosis in the absence of another source. **Hematological disorder** is defined as hemolytic anemia with reticulocytosis; leukopenia of less than 4000 white blood cells per mm^3; lymphopenia of less than 1500 lymphocytes per mm^3; or thrombocytopenia of less than 100,000 platelets per mm^3 on complete blood count on two separate occasions. **Inmunological disorder** is defined by the presence of autoantibodies to native (double-stranded) DNA, or the anti-Smith autoantibodies, or antiphospholipid antibodies [2].

What is the prevalence of SLE?

This disease is most common in women of child-bearing age of Afro-American, Afro-Caribbean, Chinese, Asian, and South American Indian ancestry. Northern Europeans are affected less often. The prevalence ranges from 40-65 per 100,000 population in Sweden and San Francisco, respectively, and higher in Afro-American women. Of interest, indigenous West Africans are less affected than their descendants living in North America or the Caribbean.

What does a positive ANA mean?

Over 95% of patients with SLE have a positive ANA, although the ANA can also be positive, albeit in low titers, <1:80, in completely normal, healthy individuals. The possibility of having a benign, positive ANA increases with age, female sex and possibly racial background. In addition, many other autoimmune diseases besides SLE are associated with a positive ANA. If positive in conjunction with an objective abnormality suggestive of lupus, then an ANA supports the diagnosis.

On the other hand, a positive ANA in association with nonspecific arthralgias and myalgias is not highly indicative of SLE [3]. Thus, an ANA is very sensitive for SLE, but it is also very nonspecific. The ANA may appear homogeneous, rim or peripheral, speckled, anticentromere, or anti-nucleolar on immunofluorescence staining. The homogeneous pattern is more likely associated with an asymptomatic state or a drug-induced condition, while the speckled staining pattern is associated with the anti-Smith antibody, anti-RNP antibody, and anti-Ro and anti-La antibodies (See chapter on clinical laboratory for more on the antinuclear antibodies). The rim or peripheral staining pattern of ANA is the most specific for active lupus nephritis, and correlates with anti-double-stranded DNA antibodies. However, immunofluorescent staining patterns are presently relied on less than in the past. The ANA is usually reported by titer. A high ANA titer, e.g., ≥1:640, is not associated with increased disease activity, but a high titer more likely represents a true positive test while a low titer ANA, e.g., ≤1:80, a false positive test.

What is the significance of some of the other autoantibodies?

The anti-Smith antibody assay is positive in up to 30% of SLE patients, but this test is very specific for the disease. The anti-double-stranded (native) DNA antibody assay is also specific for SLE, but false positive results do occur, particularly with the ELISA method. The Farr assay and *Crithidia luciliae* method of detecting anti-dsDNA antibodies are more specific for SLE. It should be said that the diagnosis of SLE is based primarily on objective evidence from the history and physical examination and not merely from the presence of certain autoantibodies.

What is the undifferentiated connective tissue syndrome?

This entity is defined as patients who do not fit criteria for any specific connective tissue disorder, but do display some objective abnormalities. Patients usually present with arthralgias or arthritis and Raynaud phenomenon and test weakly positive for rheumatoid factor or antinuclear antibody. Sometimes, there is muscle involvement, rash and fever. In some treatment centers, nearly half of rheumatology referrals are for an undifferentiated connective tissue syndrome. Nonsteroidal anti-inflammatory drugs usually suffice in controlling joint pain. Progression to a specific connective tissue syndrome can occur, such as rheumatoid arthritis, systemic lupus erythematosus, systemic sclerosis (scleroderma), or an inflammatory myopathy.

Can a patient have both rheumatoid arthritis and SLE?

SLE can occur in a patient with RA and vice versa. This combination takes the facetious appellation of "rhupus." It is important to note that objective physical signs such as rheumatoid nodules and discoid rash characterize such a syndrome, and the simultaneous presence of positive rheumatoid factor and positive ANA is not sufficient. Indeed, positive rheumatoid factor occurs in SLE, per se, and positive ANAs can be detected in RA, *per se*. It is the clinical presentation that defines the syndrome.

What treatments are available for patients with SLE?

Most lupus patients are sensitive to ultraviolet radiation and need to be cautioned about sun protection. Nonsteroidal antiinflammatory drugs can ameliorate arthritis in SLE. Antimalarials, especially hydroxychloroquine, have numerous benefits and few risks, and should be used in practically all lupus patients [(4)]. Patients treated with hydroxychloroquine have fewer lupus flares [(4)]. Furthermore, hydroxychloroquine can improve lupus arthritis, rash and fatigue. Corticosteroids are very effective but carry significant long-term risks. Any patient that requires high doses of steroid for an extended period of time should be treated with an additional agent, such as methotrexate, as a steroid sparing medication. Patients with life threatening major organ involvement (e.g., renal, neurological, pericardial, hematological) or serious vasculitis should be treated with cyclophosphamide. Intravenous, once monthly "pulse" cyclophosphamide therapy is less toxic than a daily oral regimen,and it is of proven efficacy for lupus nephritis. Furthermore, short-term induction therapy with intravenous cyclophosphamide followed by mycophenolate or azathioprine for maintenance therapy was associated with a significantly decreased incidence of chronic renal failure, adverse effects, including severe infections, and mortality compared to long-term intravenous cyclophosphamide alone [(5)].

What is on the horizon for SLE?

Newer treatments tailored to specific aspects of the pathophysiology of SLE are being studied with optimism [(6)]. B cell depletion therapy looks promising in early studies of treatment of refractory SLE. The CD20 antigen is expressed on B cells, and **rituximab**, a chimeric anti-CD20 IgG1 monoclonal antibody, depletes B cells [(7)]. In the future, mycophenolate mofetil may replace cyclophosphamide because of a wider margin of safety [(8)].

Can lupus patients have normal pregnancies?

While there is evidence that some women, particularly African-American women, develop significant lupus flares during pregnancy, some do not. Patients need to be closely monitored by their rheumatologists and obstetricians. Hypertension and /or proteinuria should be evaluated very closely[9,10]. Pregnancy is advised for patients with SLE only if there disease is in remission, or mildly active and stable without renal disease.

Can lupus patients receive estrogen replacement therapy?

Although estrogen is felt to play a role in the pathogenesis of SLE, patients may take supplemental estrogen. It is preferable to use very low doses, and the disease activity should be minimal and stable prior to therapy. The patient needs to be aware that such therapy can result in a flare of their disease activity, although this possibility is small[11].

Why are premature atherosclerosis, heart attacks and strokes more prevalent in lupus patients?

SLE is a risk factor for atherosclerotic disease. Patients with SLE have **accelerated atherosclerosis**, the consequence of inflammatory endothelial damage. The classic risk factors, diabetes mellitus, hypertension, smoking, and elevated levels of low density lipoprotein, exacerbate this problem[12, 13]. Furthermore, hyperhomocysteinemia and hypertriglyceridemia play a role in the accelerated atherosclerosis of SLE. Thus, it cannot be overemphasized that **both** aggressive coronary risk factor management and control of active lupus are important to decrease the incidence of precocious myocardial infarction and stroke in this disease.

KEY POINTS

- SLE is an autoimmune, multisystem disease affecting practically any organ in the body. Most prominently involved are the musculoskeletal system, skin, kidneys, nervous system, pleura and pericardium, and the hematological system.
- Constitutional symptoms are often prominent and include fever, loss of appetite and weight, general malaise, and easy fatigability.
- The antinuclear antibody (ANA) test is the most sensitive laboratory test for SLE, (few false negatives) and the anti-native (or double-stranded) DNA and anti-Smith antibody tests the most specific (very few false positives). However, diseases other than

SLE are also associated with ANAs (the ANA is a nonspecific test), and patients with SLE often do not have anti-native DNA or Smith antibodies (insensitive tests).

- Elevated anti-native DNA titers and decreased serum complement levels C3, C4, or CH50, correlate with active lupus nephritis. A rising anti-native DNA titer and dropping complement level can herald an exacerbation.
- Optimal control of SLE usually requires the use of hydroxychloroquine, which helps lessen flares.
- Nonsteroidal antiinflammatory drugs can control lupus arthritis, but hydroxychloroquine is beneficial in refractory cases.
- Corticosteroids are indicated for patients not responding to nonsteroidal antiinflammatory drugs or hydroxychloroquine, or for patients with vital organ involvement.
- Intravenous pulse or oral cyclophosphamide is indicated for lupus nephritis or other life-threatening manifestations of SLE. Intravenous, pulse therapy is generally less toxic.
- Other drugs such as methotrexate, azathioprine, dihydroepiandrostendione (DHEA), mycophenolate mofetil, and leflunomide play a role in the therapy of some patients with SLE as well. Mycophenolate mofetil, in particular, will have an important function in SLE in the near future.
- Due to the precocious coronary artery disease lupus patients develop, vigorous efforts to ameliorate reversible coronary risks factors should be undertaken. Similarly vaccinations for influenza and pneumococcal disease are very important.
- The prognosis of SLE has generally improved over the past few decades.

CHAPTER 9

THE ANTIPHOSPHOLIPID SYNDROME (HUGHES SYNDROME)

Harold M Adelman

What is the Antiphospholipid (APL) syndrome?

At a recent meeting in Sydney, Australia, the classification criteria for definite antiphospholipid syndrome were re-formulated. There must be at least one clinical and one laboratory criterion present. Clinically, essentially, venous or arterial thrombosis and/or loss of a morphologically normal fetus at or beyond the 10th week of pregnancy; laboratory criteria include plasma lupus anticoagulant on two or more occasions at least 12 weeks apart; IgG or IGM anticardiolipin antibodies greater than 40 GPL or MPL, on two or more occasions at least 12 weeks apart; IgG and/or IgM anti-beta2-glycoprotein 1 antibodies present on two or more occasions, at least 12 weeks apart. (Miyakis S, Lockchin, MD, Atsumi T, et al. International consensus statement on the update of the Classification Criteria for definite antiphospholipid syndrome [APS]. J Thomb & Haemost 2006;4:295-306.) One can see livedo reticularis in this syndrome (Figure 1).

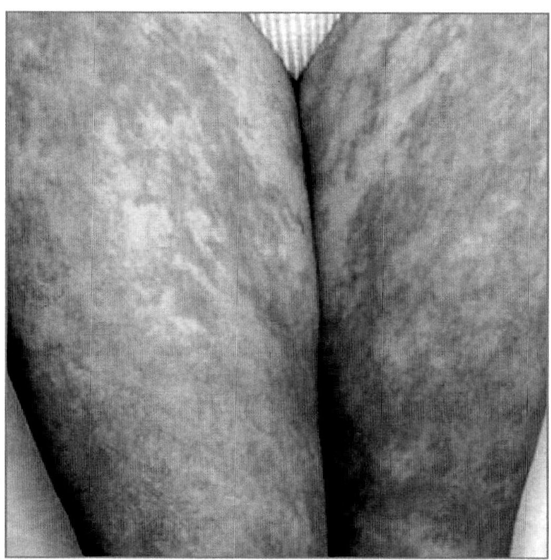

Figure 1. *Severe livedo reticularis of the legs. This condition is a net-like, purple discoloration on the extremities and can be present in any of the diffuse connective tissue diseases.*
Doria A, Rondinone R, University of Padova, Italy

How is the diagnosis of this syndrome made?

Diagnosis is based on the presence of one clinical and one laboratory criterion. The laboratory criterion should be positive on more than one occasion, at least 12 weeks apart. The more criteria present, the more likely would be the diagnosis of antiphospholipid syndrome [1, 2].

What are antiphospholipid antibodies?

Antiphospholipid antibodies bind to the antigen beta2 –glycoprotein-1 (ß2GP1). ß2GP1 is a naturally occurring phospholipid-binding protein. Cardiolipin antibodies and the lupus anticoagulant are both antiphospholipid antibodies. The term lupus anticoagulant can be a source of confusion, as many patients with this autoantibody do not have lupus, and it is an anticoagulant *in vitro* only; it is a procoagulant *in vivo*.

What is the pathogenesis of this syndrome?

Several mechanisms can explain the antiphospholipid syndrome. ß2GP1 acts as an anticoagulant by inhibiting the contact activation of the coagulation sequence and also the conversion of prothrombin to thrombin. In fact, the lupus anticoagulant prolongs the activated partial thromboplastin time when added to normal serum but not when added to plasma depleted of beta2-glycoprotein 1. Thus, by binding and neutralizing ß2GP1, antiphospholipid antibodies induce thrombosis. Antiphospholipid antibodies also interfere with protein C activation, thus causing a hypercoagulable state.

What are the primary and secondary antiphospholipid syndromes?

In the absence of an inciting disease, the syndrome is called the primary antiphospholipid syndrome. When the antiphospholipid syndrome is induced by another disease, it is called secondary. Examples of inciting diseases are other autoimmune diseases, especially systemic lupus erythematosus, malignancies, and infections.

What are the principle clinical features of the antiphospholipid syndrome?

Deep venous thrombosis with pulmonary embolism is a cardinal feature of the APS syndrome. Venous thrombosis also occur in the hepatic vein, causing the Budd-Chiari syndrome, renal vein, axillary, subclavian, and retinal veins as well as the vena cavae. Aggravating events, such as a long trip, surgery, taking estrogen-containing oral contraceptives, or smoking can elicit thrombosis in a patient predisposed by antiphospholipid antibodies. An elevated anticardiolipin antibody titer six months after venous thromboembolism is a strong predictor of recurrence and death. The risk correlates with titer. Prolonged anticoagulation is indicated for these patients[3].

Arterial thrombosis can cause stroke, amaurosis fugax, myocardial infarction, peripheral gangrene, or bowel infarction. When they recur, the same kind of thrombosis usually occurs in the same individual, that is, venous or arterial. **Recurrent abortions** are probably the result of placental infarcts and occur in any trimester. **Thrombocytopenia** is occasionally severe.

The site of thrombosis might be related to the type of autoantibody: Venous thromboembolic disease is usually caused by the lupus anticoagulant; and cerebral, coronary, and peripheral arterial thrombosis is usually caused by anticardiolipin antibodies. Furthermore, antibody specificity likely influences risk of thrombosis, that is, antibodies to beta-2-glycoprotein 1 and antiphospholipids is likely more thrombophilic than antibodies to either alone. Higher antibody titer is another thrombosis risk factor.

What are the best methods of detecting anticardiolipin antibodies and the lupus anticoagulant?

An ELISA method is used to detect anticardiolipin antibodies. Ten percent bovine serum containing ß2GP1 is necessary for a valid test. Results are reported by titer and isotype, IgG in GPL (G phospholipid) units, and IgM in MPL (M phospholipid) units.

The activated partial thromboplastin test is used as a screening test for the lupus anticoagulant. Another test should then be positive to diagnose the presence of these autoantibodies, such as the Russell viper venom time or the kaolin clotting time. The presence of the lupus anticoagulant is also confirmed when the prolonged aPTT is shortened or normalized by adding excess phospholipid, or the aPTT persists prolonged when the patient's plasma is mixed with normal, platelet poor plasma – barring a clotting factor deficiency.

What is the best way to manage the antiphospholipid syndrome?

As arterial or venous thromboses tend to recur, indefinite warfarin therapy is indicated [4]. The benefit of thrombosis prevention is much higher than the incidence of bleeding. It should be pointed out, however, that not all studies support this finding. A minor thrombosis in the calf might not require indefinite anticoagulation, though indefinite aspirin use would be recommended. A single, major thrombosis, such as a pulmonary embolism or hepatic vein thrombosis, on the other hand, is an indication for lifelong anticoagulation in the antiphospholipid syndrome. The optimal INR for the antiphospholipid syndome is being clarified. Some authors recommend an INR between 3.1 and 3.5, others an INR between 2.0 and 3.0. [5, 6]. A recent article questions the need to anticoagulate patients with a first ischemic stroke, at least if antiphospholipid antibodies are tested for only once soon after the stroke [7].

A caveat about acetaminophen: This medication can enhance warfarin's effect [8]. Therefore, the INR level needs to be monitored more often when acetaminophen is added to a patient's regimen at doses above 1.3 g/day for more than a week. Another problem monitoring the INR is when the antiphospholipid antibodies have anti-prothrombin activity, prolonging the INR. In this situation, measurement of the chromogenic factor X level or the prothrombin-proconvertin time in lieu of the INR is helpful. It is interesting to note that in a controlled trial, Watzke et al found that patients who monitored their own INR weekly at home achieved a therapeutic INR more often than those who had their INR monitored conventionally at an Anticoagulation Clinic [9].

What about the patient found to have antiphospholipid antibodies who has never had a thrombosis?

These patients do not have to be treated prophylactically with warfarin. However, a patient with high levels of antiphospholipid antibodies should be treated with an aspirin tablet a day. Also, oral birth control pills ought to be avoided in patients with antiphospholipid antibodies.

Are there situations requiring special consideration?

In cases of widespread, life-threatening thromboses, the so-called "catastrophic antiphospholipid syndrome", not responding to warfarin, the use of immunosuppressives, plasmapheresis, fibrinolytics, or intravenous gamma globulin has helped some patients. For prophylaxis for general surgery, give

5000 units of unfractionated heparin subcutaneously one hour before the procedure. For orthopedic procedures, give low molecular weight heparin. If there is no bleeding post operatively, restart warfarin.

How are women with recurrent miscarriages managed?

As warfarin is teratogenic , use low molecular weight heparin subcutaneously. For example, enoxaparin 40 mg daily until 12 weeks of gestation, then 40 mg twice daily. As even low molecular weight heparin can cause osteoporosis, adequate calcium, 1500 mg a day, and vitamin D 800 IU a day, are important. In patients to receive regional anesthesia at delivery, a switch to unfractionated heparin near anticipated delivery is important to avoid an epidural hematoma. The effect of unfractionated heparin is shorter than that of low molecular weight heparin and easier to terminate. Postpartum, continue enoxaparin, 40 mg subcutaneously twice daily for 12 weeks. Some authorities suggest one 81mgm aspirin tablet a day with low molecular weight heparin [10, 11].

How do you treat severe thrombocytopenia, <20,000 per mm^3, in the antiphospholipid syndrome?

Life-threatening thrombocytopenia, although not common, occurs and is treated with corticosteroids, immunosuppressives, or intravenous gamma globulin. For the dilemma of a patient with thromboses and severe thrombocytopenia, for whom anticoagulation can cause major bleeding, it is advisable to get the platelet count over 50,000 per mm^3 with glucocorticoids or intravenous immunoglobulin before resuming anticoagulation [12]. Moreover, it is important to remember that heparin itself can cause a life-threatening, immune thrombocytopenia, "HIT," or heparin-induced thrombocytopenia, and "the white clot syndrome" with paradoxical thromboses.

KEY POINTS

- The antiphospholipid syndrome is a hypercoagulable state characterized clinically by venous and arterial thromboses, and recurrent abortions.
- Laboratory features include thrombocytopenia, the lupus anticoagulant and/or anticardiolipin antibodies.

- The antiphospholipid syndrome can be primary, or secondary to other rheumatic diseases, especially systemic lupus erythematosus, malignancies, or infections.
- The term lupus anticoagulant is a misnomer, as it is really a procoagulant in vivo, and many patients with this antibody do not have lupus.
- An important protein in the pathogenesis of this syndrome is ß2-glycoprotein 1 (ß2GP1). This protein is itself an anticoagulant, and antiphospholipid antibodies may induce thrombosis by neutralizing ß2GP1.
- While currently being clarified, anticoagulant treatment of the antiphospholipid syndrome requires warfarin dosed to an INR around 2.5.

CHAPTER 10

SJÖGREN SYNDROME

Harold M Adelman

What is Sjögren syndrome (SS)?

Sjögren syndrome (SS) is a multisystem autoimmune disease, principally affecting exocrine glands and characterized clinically by the so-called sicca complex of dry eyes – keratoconjunctivitis sicca and dry mouth – xerostomia. Occasionally, there are enlarged salivary glands and other exocrine gland involvement [(1)]. SS can be primary, or secondary to other autoimmune diseases, such as rheumatoid arthritis, systemic sclerosis (scleroderma), systemic lupus erythematosus, and polymyositis. Secondary SS also accompanies autoimmune disorders not in the realm of the "connective tissue disease," such as thyroiditis, primary biliary cirrhosis, and multiple sclerosis [(2)]. This discussion will concern primary SS. Recently, the American-European Consensus Group modified the classification criteria for Sjogren's syndrome [(3)].

How prevalent is this condition?

SS is second to rheumatoid arthritis as the most common autoimmune rheumatic disease. Approximately 1% of the US population has Sjögren's syndrome. In the UK and Greece, approximately 3.5% of people over 65 years of age, and in Sweden, 2.7% have primary Sjögren syndrome. It is ten times more common in women, likely a consequence of the effect of sex hormones on the immune system. Rheumatoid arthritis is the most commonly associated connective tissue disease in secondary Sjogren syndrome with about 20% of RA patients having clinical manifestations of Sjogren syndrome.

What is the pathogenesis of this disorder?

There is disordered lymphocyte regulation. Various exocrine glands are invaded by CD4+ T cells, and to a lesser degree B cells, with consequent tissue destruction [(1)]. IgA-bearing plasma cells also play a role in the pathogenesis of SS. In addition, abnormalities of apoptosis, programmed cell death, are prominent in the pathogenesis of this syndrome. Abnormal apoptosis involves infiltrating mononuclear cells and epithelial cells, affecting presentation of autoantigens to T cells. This fact, interestingly, can explain the abnormal salivary or lacrimal gland function that takes place even before there is prominent lymphocyte infiltration [2]. Enhanced expression of Fas, a cell surface protein whose ligation triggers apoptosis in lymphocytes and in fibroblasts, and DNA strand breaks, an indication of cell death, are seen in ductal epithelium and acinar cells of salivary and lacrimal glands [4]. Indeed, accelerated apoptosis causes exposure of nuclear antigens to the immune system. Moreover, persistence of autoimmune T cell clones from faulty apoptosis heightens their attack against self. Perhaps interplay between latent viruses tropic for exocrine glands, e.g., the Epstein –Barr virus, and aberrant apoptosis combine to produce chronic target tissue inflammation. A better comprehension of abnormal apoptotic mechanisms will allow more effective therapy.

Is there evidence of humeral autoimmunity in Sjögren's syndrome?

IgG against muscarinic M3 receptors have been found in the serum of patients with Sjögren's syndrome. Secretagogues such as pilocarpine and cevimeline stimulate saliva secretion by stimulating muscarinic receptors, and may be effective in SS by competing with anti-muscarinic 3 antibodies. These agents must be used with much caution in patients with asthma, narrow-angle glaucoma, severe cardiovascular disease, biliary tree disease, and peptic ulcer disease because they also stimulate muscarinic activity in other organs.

Which cytokines are important in the pathogenesis of Sjögren's syndrome?

Tumor necrosis factor-alpha, interleukin–2 and 6 as well as interferon-gamma are prominent cytokines in Sjögren's syndrome. Interferon-gamma expression appears to discriminate between SS and healthy controls [5].

What are some clinical features suggestive of the keratoconjunctivitis of SS?

There is an annoying foreign-body sensation that gets worse as the day progresses. However, a history of eye pain and photophobia is more indicative of anterior uveitis.

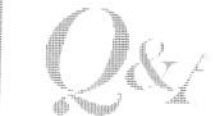

What are the oral and ocular complications of SS?

Rampant dental caries, angular cheilitis from candida infection, filamentary keratitis, corneal abrasion and infections can be consequences of xerostomia and keratoconjunctivitis sicca.

What are the sour ball sign and the cracker sign?

Patients with SS and an intolerably dry mouth tend to suck sour balls for relief. They should be instructed to use sugarless candy because of their susceptibility to rampant caries. In addition, these patients will tell you they cannot swallow dry crackers (because of the paucity of saliva). Such patients walk around with a water bottle.

What other conditions can cause enlargement of the salivary glands?

Sarcoidosis, tumors, amyloidosis, iodide sensitivity, excessive alcohol ingestion, and infections, e.g., tuberculosis, syphilis, and human immunodeficiency virus infection – so called DILS (Figure 1), or the diffuse infiltrative lymphocytosis syndrome – can also cause enlargement of the salivary glands[(6)].

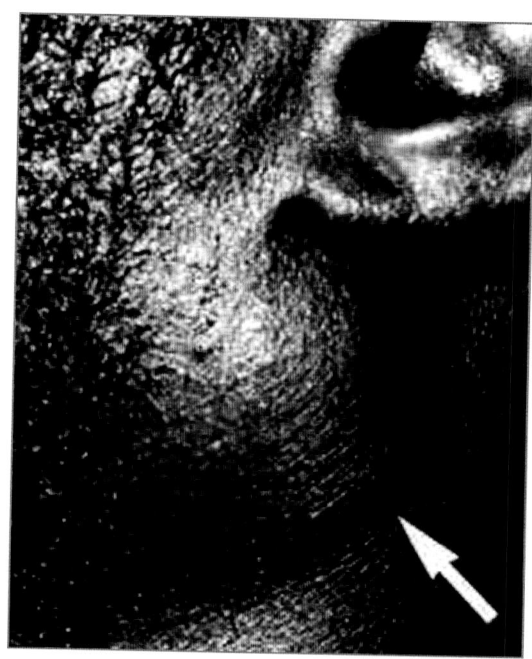

Figure 1. *The left parotid gland of this man with AIDS is swollen (arrow) from DILS, which is clinically indistinguishable from Sjogren syndrome.*

Reprinted with kind permission of JAMA .Schrot RJ, Adelman HM, Linden CN, Wallach PM. Cystic parotid gland enlargement in HIV disease. The diffuse infiltrative lymphocytosis syndrome. JAMA 1997;278:166-7.

What other organ involvement can occur in SS?

The mucosa of the upper airways, lungs, and vagina, and the skin, kidneys, gastrointestinal system, and nervous system can be involved in SS. Clinical manifestations of such involvement include dryness of the upper airways and lungs, bronchitis, lymphocytic interstitial pneumonitis, pseudolymphoma and non-Hodgkin's lymphoma, and pleuritis with or without effusions. Vaginal dryness causes discomfort, dyspareunia and infection. Women with Sjögren syndrome can have symptoms of cystitis, such as dysuria, urinary frequency, urgency, and nocturia. Xerosis, dry skin, can be quite bothersome. Cutaneous vasculitis is a feature of Sjögren syndrome. Kidney involvement leads to tubulointerstitial nephritis with type I renal tubular acidosis. Hypokalemic periodic paralysis can ensue. Lymphoma and renal artery vasculitis are other renal manifestations of Sjogren's syndrome. Gastrointestinal involvement from lack of saliva or atrophic gastritis, and biliary cirrhosis is a concomitant.

In addition, constitutional symptoms, such as fatigue, fever, and myalgias, occur in SS, and Raynaud phenomenon is also seen. Sometimes, there is frank arthritis or systemic vasculitis. Thyroiditis with hypothyroidism occurs in about 15% of patients with SS, and anemia, leukopenia, and thrombocytopenia can be present.

What is the nervous system involvement in SS?

Neurological disease is one of the most significant extraglandular manifestations of SS. Nervous system involvement can be central or peripheral and can cause a multiple sclerosis-like picture, mononeuritis multiplex, or symmetric involvement of the hands and feet, with ataxia. Sural nerve biopsies show vasculitis of the vasa nervorum in some cases. Autonomic neuropathy can cause orthostatic hypotension. There can be cranial nerve involvement, especially trigeminal neuropathy. Sensorineural hearing loss involving high-pitched frequencies is not uncommon in SS[7]. Transverse myelopathy can occur in neuro-SS. This medical emergency is treated with glucocorticoids and cyclophosphamide[2]. Cognitive dysfunction is seen, and SS patients often develop fatigue and fibromyalgia.

What are the diagnostic criteria of SS?

The diagnostic criteria[8] include:

- Symptoms and objective signs of ocular dryness, including a Schirmer's test and Rose Bengal staining of the cornea. Wetting of less than 5 mm in five minutes of a filter paper placed in the inferior conjunctival sac constitutes

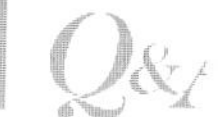

a positive Schirmer's test. Rose Bengal staining of the cornea indicates keratoconjunctivitis sica.

- Symptoms and objective signs of dry mouth, such as decreased parotid flow rate using Lashley cups and an abnormal minor salivary gland (lip) biopsy, with an average focal, periductal lymphocyte infiltrate of >50 lymphocytes per 4 mm^2 of four evaluable lobules
- The presence of autoantibodies, such as rheumatoid factor >1:160, antinuclear antibody >1;160, and presence of anti-SS-A (Ro) or anti-SSB (La) antibodies.

A definite diagnosis of SS is made if items one, two and an autoantibody are present. Probable SS is diagnosed in the absence of a minor salivary gland biopsy. For the diagnosis of SS, certain conditions must be excluded, such as sarcoidosis, pre-existing lymphoma, AIDS, other causes of salivary gland enlargement, or dysautonomia. The importance of a careful diagnosis lies in the importance of excluding a treatable SS mimic, such as use of an anticholinergic medication.

What conditions should be considered in the differential diagnosis of SS?

Clinically, sarcoidosis can look like SS, with salivary gland swelling, dry eyes, dry mouth, and arthritis. The presence of anterior uveitis, and noncaseating granulomas on biopsy distinguish sarcoidosis from SS. Graft-versus-host disease after bone marrow transplantation can include the sicca complex. Although biopsy specimens look more like severe lichen planus, the history of a bone marrow transplant clarifies the picture. Radiation to the head and neck can be followed by the sicca complex, and sometimes the dry eyes and mouth may follow years after radiation. Some patients with HIV disease get enlarged salivary glands with dry eyes and mouth. Biopsy shows an infiltrate consisting of CD8 cells, instead of the CD4 cells of SS. This condition in HIV disease is called DILS, for Diffuse Infiltrative Lymphocytosis Syndrome [9]. The presence of HIV disease and the CD8 lymphocyte infiltrate make the distinction from SS. Other conditions that cause enlargement of the parotid glands are mentioned above.

When should a minor salivary gland biopsy be performed?

If an alternative cause of salivary gland enlargement, such as sarcoidosis or lymphoma, is suspected, a minor salivary gland biopsy is indicated [10].

What is the risk of non-Hodgkin's lymphoma in patients with SS?

Patients with SS have 40 times the risk of non-Hodgkin's lymphoma of age and sex-matched general population controls[11]. These lymphomas are principally B cell in origin, and often involve mucosa-associated lymphoid tissue – MALT lymphomas. Extranodal sites are often involved and include the salivary glands, gastrointestinal tract, the lung, kidney, skin, thymus and thyroid gland[2].

What are anti-SSA (Sjögren syndrome A) and anti-SSB (Sjögren syndrome B) antibodies?

Anti-SSA, also called anti-Ro antibodies, are IgG antibodies against a 60 or 52 kD protein associated with small cellular RNAs. Anti-SSB, also called anti-La antibodies, are IgG antibodies against a 48 kD phosphoprotein complexed with RNA polymerase III transcripts. These antigens reside in the nucleus. They are seen primarily in SS and systemic lupus erythematosus. The sensitivity of anti- SSA (anti-Ro) antibodies for primary SS is up to 70%, and for systemic lupus erythematosus 30%. The sensitivity of anti-SSB (anti-La) antibodies for primary SS is about up to 60%, and for systemic lupus erythematosus, 15%.

Is there an HLA haplotype correlation of these autoantibodies?

Anti-SS-A and B autoantibodies correlate with the HLA-B8-DR3 haplotype in Caucasians.

How is SS managed?

The dry eyes are treated with a hydroxymethylcellulose, a polymer-like dextran-based artificial tear product. Different preparations might have to be tried before the patient finds a satisfactory product. Punctal occlusion sometimes is necessary to block tear drainage. The aim is to keep the eyes moist to avoid corneal abrasion and infection. Topical ophthalmic cyclosporin emulsion has recently been approved for use.

For the dry mouth, sugarless hard candy or gum, and sugarless mints can be helpful, as can artificial saliva. However, other carbohydrates in these products also can cause dental caries in people with reduced saliva. Chewing on paraffin wax or a fruit pit might suffice. Oral pilocarpine has been added to the armamentarium. A 5 mg tablet four times a day improves dry mouth and eyes as well as other xeroses[12]. Oral yeast infection and angular cheilitis is treated with nystatin swish and swallow or a topical antifungal, respectively.

Central heating or air conditioning can exacerbate the sicca symptoms, and a humidifier often helps.

Arthralgias are treated with NSAIDs, hydroxychloroquine, and/or low dose prednisone. For vasculitis, pneumonitis, neuropathy or nephritis, corticosteroids are employed and cyclophosphamide can be effective in life-threatening disease. However, since patients with SS are susceptible to lymphoma, it is important to be on the alert for this malignancy, and cyclophosphamide should be used in the pulse intravenous format rather than a daily oral regimen. In recent studies, tumor necrosis factor alpha blocker therapy looks promising (13). Finally, patients with SS who undergo surgery are at risk of certain complications, such as pneumonia, and the anesthesiologist must be aware that the patient has SS.

What is the prognosis for patients with SS?

Most patients with SS do well with optimal management. However, some of the associated diseases, such as lymphoma, may complicate the prognosis. One in five deaths in primary SS is from lymphoma. Predictive factors are palpable cutaneous purpura and a low C4 level at presentation. A hardened parotid is suggestive of lymphoma of this gland (14). Other signposts for lymphoma are the development of a monoclonal protein, new-onset leukopenia or anemia, and loss of previously attendant autoantibodies, such as rheumatoid factor, antinuclear antibodies or SS-A or B (2). Patients with Sjögren syndrome should be followed by a physician with experience in this disease.

KEY POINTS

- The Sjögren syndrome (the sicca syndrome, with xerostomia and keratoconjunctivitis sicca) is an autoimmune exocrinopathy with a predilection for the lacrimal and salivary glands. Lymphocytes infiltrate and destroy glandular parenchyma.
- This syndrome can be primary, or secondary to another autoimmune disease, most often rheumatoid arthritis.
- Fifty percent of patients with secondary Sjögren syndrome have rheumatoid arthritis. Looked at the other way, 20% of patients with rheumatoid arthritis have Sjögren syndrome.

- Other rheumatic diseases associated with Sjögren syndrome are systemic sclerosis (scleroderma) and systemic lupus erythematosus.
- The clinical hallmarks of Sjögren syndrome are dry eyes and dry mouth. Patients can have rampant dental caries and develop upper airways diseases such as bronchitis. Other manifestations are dry skin and dry vaginal mucosa with dyspareunia.
- Vasculitis and arthritis are also seen in primary Sjögren syndrome.
- Low-grade B cell lymphoma is seen with significantly increased frequency in patients with Sjögren syndrome. The cervical lymph nodes and salivary glands are particularly predisposed.
- Treatment of the sicca symptoms is centered around artificial tears and artificial saliva.
- Hydroxychloroquine is helpful for arthralgias, myalgias and lymphadenopathy, and glucocorticoids are indicated for vasculitis.
- Cyclophosphamide, used for life threatening, systemic SS, must be used with special caution because of the tendency to lymphoma in Sjögren syndrome. If essential for life-threatening Sjögren syndrome, cyclophosphamide should be administered as pulse therapy rather than daily oral therapy. Rheumatology consultation is warranted.

CHAPTER 11

IDIOPATHIC INFLAMMATORY MYOPATHIES

Keith D Kanik

What are the idiopathic inflammatory myopathies?

The idiopathic inflammatory myopathies include the following: primary polymyositis and dermatomyositis, dermatomyositis associated with malignancy, childhood polymyositis or dermatomyositis, polymyositis or dermatomyositis associated with another connective tissue disease, inclusion body myositis, and miscellaneous inflammatory myopathies (e.g., eosinophilic myositis). Practically pathognomonic of dermatomyositis are the heliotrope rash of the eyelids (Figure 1, left panel) and Gottron's sign (Figure 1, right panel). The heliotrope suffusion of the eyelids is a lilac-colored rash that resembles the hue of the heliotrope rose [1]. Gottron's sign is a scaly, macular rash over the knuckles. There can also be Gottron's papules over the knuckles.

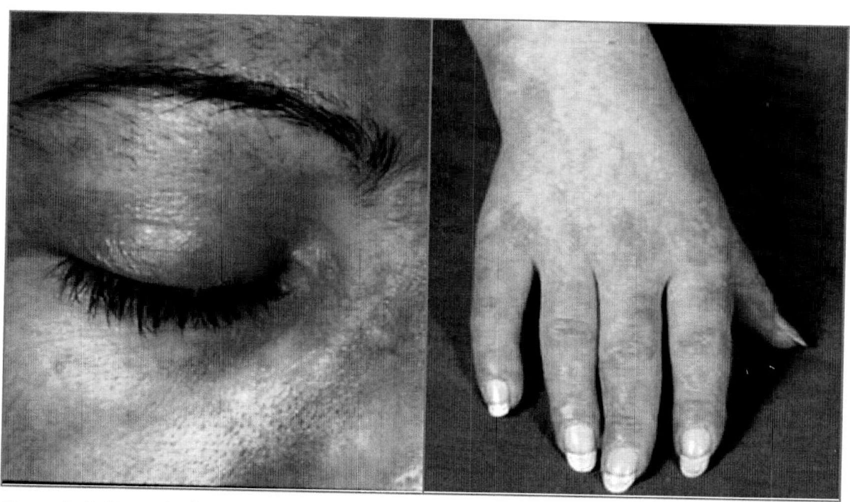

Figure 1. *Left panel: This patient with dermatomyositis demonstrates the periorbital heliotrope rash of dermatomyositis.* *Grassi, W, University of Ancona, Italy.*

Right panel: The Gottron sign of dermatomyositis is a scaly, macular rash over the knuckles. *Taggard, A at Musgrave Park Hospital, Belfast.*

What are the clinical signs of myositis?

Symmetrical proximal muscle weakness is the hallmark of this group of diseases. Proximal muscle groups include shoulder and hip girdle muscles - that is, the neck flexors and extensors and the deltoids, the hip flexors and extensors, and quadriceps. Inclusion body myositis, an under-recognized disease, is exceptional in that it typically manifests as proximal and distal muscle weakness.

What is the prevalence of polymyositis and dermatomyositis?

This disease occurs in all parts of the world, and the prevalence ranges from 2.4 to 10.7 cases per 100,000 population. It is more common in black people. Polymyositis is seen twice as often as dermatomyositis.

How is myositis diagnosed?

Proximal muscle weakness, elevated muscle enzymes (particularly creatine kinase), myopathic electromyography, and an abnormal muscle biopsy allow diagnosis. Pathologic findings on biopsy are degenerating and regenerating muscle fibers, centralization of nuclei and a lymphocytic infiltrate. There is also, absence of histological changes of another myopathy.

What should be in the differential diagnosis of the idiopathic inflammatory myopathies?

There are many diseases that mimic myositis. Drugs can cause myopathy, including colchicine, hydroxychloroquine, cyclosporine, the statins, zidovudine, alcohol and cocaine. A careful history will reveal the possibility of drug-induced myopathy. It is also important to rule out endocrine and electrolyte disorders, particularly hypokalemia, hypomagnesemia, hypothyroidism, hyperthyroidism, Cushing syndrome, and Addison disease. Neuromuscular disorders, diagnosed with electro-physiologic testing, and metabolic myopathies, e.g., McArdle's disease - from muscle phosphorylase deficiency, DiMauro's disease from carnitine palmitoyltransferase deficiency, and others should also be in the differential diagnosis. Muscle biopsy with histochemical analysis will allow a diagnosis of metabolic myopathy.

Is there an association between dermatomyositis and polymyositis and malignancy?

It is important to consider malignancy in dermatomyositis and polymyositis as the occurrence of malignancy is increased in these diseases. About 15% of patients with dermatomyositis have a malignancy, and the myopathy is considered to be a paraneoplastic syndrome in these patients. The most common neoplasms generally for age and sex are those seen most often in dermatomyositis. A careful history and physical examination, a chest X-ray and the recommended health maintenance screening should be done if not up-to-date (mammogram, colonoscopy, pelvic exam, Pap smear, rectal exam and prostrate specific antigen). A more directed search for malignancy might then be performed based upon the findings [(2)]. Be particularly vigilant for cancer of the ovary, lung, or stomach. Women with dermato or polymyositis should have a trans-vaginal ultrasound scan and a blood test for the tumor marker CA 125.

Is there a laboratory test for myositis?

Besides creatine kinase (CK), myositis specific autoantibodies may be found in patients with myositis. The best defined are the anti-Jo-1 antibodies, which are associated with the antisynthetase syndrome (myositis, interstitial lung disease, Raynaud's phenomenon, arthritis, mechanic's hands, fever). Other antibodies in the IIMs include anti-SRP (signal recognition particle) and anti MI-2 antibodies. These antibodies also have clinical correlations. It should be noted that an absence of these or any autoantibodies does not preclude a diagnosis of myositis [(3)].

What is inclusion body myositis?

Sporadic inclusion body myositis (IBM) is an increasingly recognized idiopathic inflammatory myopathy (IIM) with the following characteristics:

- Clinically, there is a **neuromyopathic** picture with **distal** as well as proximal weakness. There is muscle atrophy.
- Deep tendon reflexes are decreased.
- There is absence of rash.
- There is absence of underlying malignancy.
- CK levels range from normal to 10X normal. This degree of elevation is generally less than in polymyositis or dermatomyositis.
- EMG shows both a myopathic *and* neuropathic pattern.
- In most cases, muscle biopsy shows **basophilic rimmed vacuoles and eosinophilic inclusions** on microscopy in the sarcoplasm. There are

characteristic **filamentous inclusions and vacuoles** on electron microscopy in 90% of cases.

- Some of the filaments bind to antibodies to ß-amyloid and prion proteins.
- There is a fair to poor response to glucocorticoid therapy in IBM.

What is the best way to treat myositis?

The IIMs, besides inclusion body myositis, usually respond to the early institution of glucocorticoids alone [4, 5]. Prednisone or prednisolone, 1 mg per kilogram per day, is usually employed and tapered as response permits. For patients not responding to a corticosteroid after about six weeks, methotrexate or azathioprine should be added. It is important to note, long-term steroids may often cause steroid myopathy that is difficult to differentiate from myositis. In patients with IIM responding to glucocorticoids, serum CK levels are decreasing or normal. The addition or substitution of methotrexate and/or azathioprine as a steroid-sparing agent is recommended for those cases requiring long-term glucocorticoids. Hydroxychloroquine is helpful for the treatment of a resistant rash. Cyclosporin or intravenous immunoglobulins may be considered if other therapies fail [6]. If patients do not respond to treatment, an underlying malignancy is possible or the diagnosis of IIM should be reconsidered. Metabolic myopathies, such as McArdle's disease, are difficult to differentiate from myositis, and do not usually respond to immunosuppression. Biopsy with histochemical analysis will be telling.

Do patients get better?

Once muscle is destroyed it does not regenerate. With early, proper medical therapy and rehabilitation, however, patients may come close to their premorbid state.

KEY POINTS

- The clinical hallmark of the IIMs is proximal muscle weakness. Muscle pain occurs less often.
- Dermatomyositis is associated with various rashes, the most characteristic of which are a heliotrope (lilac) suffusion around the eyelids and an erythematous scaly rash over the knuckles, Gottron's sign, or Gottron's papules.

- A definite diagnosis of polymyositis is made by the presence of proximal muscle weakness, elevated muscle enzymes -- most often creatine kinase -- a myopathic electromyogram, and a muscle biopsy showing degenerating and regenerating muscle fibers, centralization of nuclei and a lymphocytic infiltrate. There is absence of histological findings of another myopathy.
- An elevated CK is the most common muscle enzyme abnormality, but in some cases an elevated aldolase in the only clue. Remember that AST and ALT are also muscle enzymes and may be elevated in myositis patients with no liver disease.
- In some series, dermatomyositis is associated with malignancy in about 15% of cases. Dermatomyositis, and less often polymyositis, is associated with malignancies common for age and sex, and standard screening, e.g., breast examination, mammogram, pelvic examination, Pap smear, colonoscopy, and rectal exam and prostrate specific antigen assay, are warranted. A chest X-ray and urinalysis should be done as well. A thorough history and physical examination and routine laboratory tests will direct any further testing.
- The treatment of polymyositis and dermatomyositis consists of a corticosteroid, such as prednisone or prednisolone, 1 mg per kilogram per day and tapered as response permits. For patients not responding to a corticosteroid after about six weeks, methotrexate or azathioprine should be added.
- Beware of ovarian cancer.

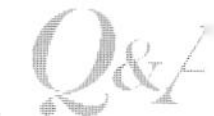

CHAPTER 12

SYSTEMIC SCLEROSIS (SCLERODERMA)

Edward P Cutolo

What is the definition of Systemic Sclerosis?

Systemic sclerosis (SSc), which literally means hard (skleros) skin (derma), is a chronic disease that affects multiple organ systems. Inflammatory, degenerative and fibrotic changes of the skin (Figure 1), blood vessels, joints, tendons, skeletal muscle, heart, lung, kidney and gastrointestinal tract occur.

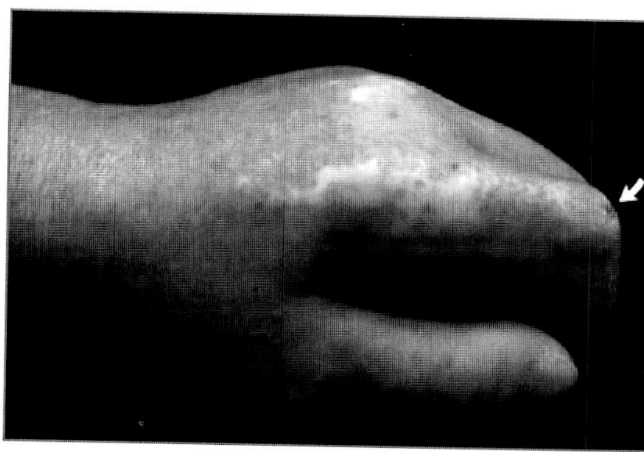

Figure 1. *The fingers of the left hand of this patient with systemic sclerosis demonstrate tight skin - sclerodactyly, hypo- and hyperpigmentation – so called salt and pepper sign, and a small ulcer on the proximal interphalangeal joint [arrow], the consequence of poorly vascularized skin.*
Grassi, W, University of Ancona, Italy.

What are the epidemiological characteristics of systemic sclerosis?

The incidence of SSc in the United States is approximately 20 new cases per one million population annually, and in the UK, 18 per million per year. Prevalence has been estimated at 125 to 250 per million. The peak age is from age 40 to 60, with a female to male ratio of 3:1. Black people are affected somewhat more frequently than whites although the incidence of SSc is higher in African-Americans than in Nigerian blacks [1, 2].

What are the classifications of the different forms of scleroderma?

In limited scleroderma, patients have cutaneous thickening of the limbs distal to the elbows, although some classifications state distal to the wrists or MCPs[3] no truncal involvement but there may be facial involvement. In diffuse scleroderma (systemic sclerosis), cutaneous thickening occurs on the distal and proximal limbs, as well as the face and trunk (Figure 2).

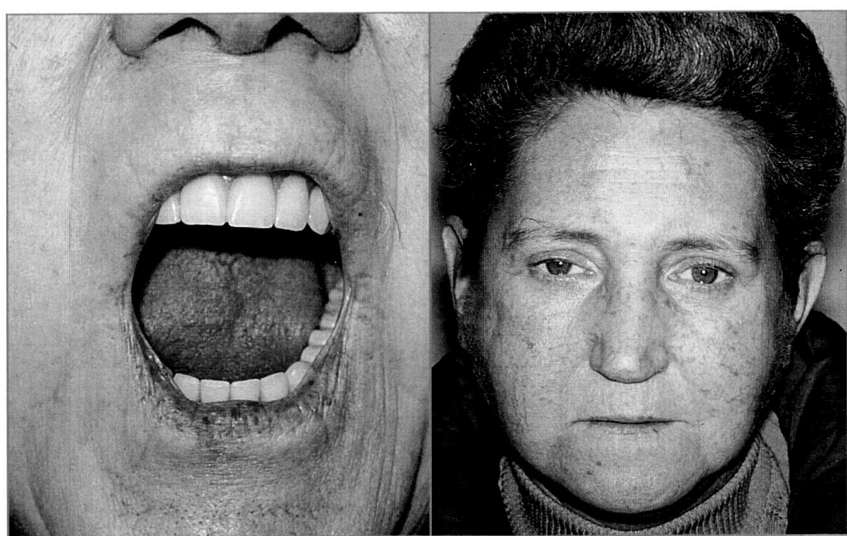

Figure 2. *Left panel: One should suspect the diagnosis of SSc walking into the room of this patient. She has tight skin and lips as well as facial telangiectasias and a limited buccal aperture.*

Right panel. This patient's facial appearance resembles that of a mouse, and is called the Mouskopf appearance.

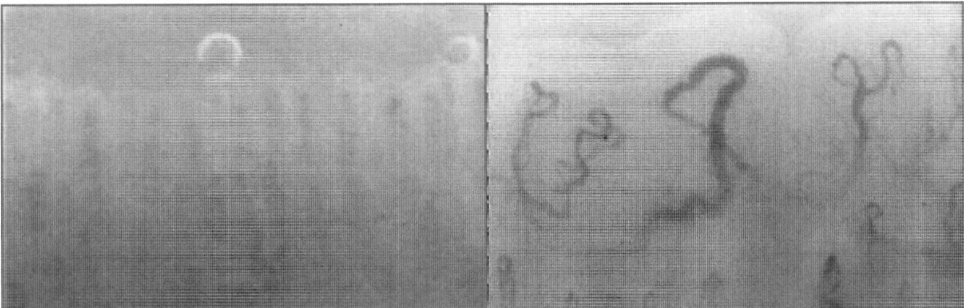

Figure 3. *Left panel: Normal capillaroscopy. Magnified 200X. Right panel: The nail fold capillaries in this patient with systemic sclerosis are dilated, with interspersed "drop out" areas without capillaries. Magnified 200X.*

Cutolo, M, Sulli A, Pizzorni C. University of Genova, Italy

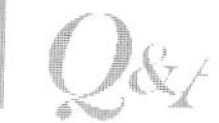

As opposed to patients with limited scleroderma, those with diffuse scleroderma have a shorter time interval between the onset of Raynaud's syndrome and significant involvement of internal organs [4]. One example is the so-called wide mouthed diverticula of the colon, which are characteristic of colon involvement in systemic sclerosis. Nail fold capillaroscopy can assist in early diagnosis of systemic sclerosis Fig. 3.

Localized scleroderma involves a patch of skin, limb or part of the face. An example is morphea.

Where does the CREST syndrome fit in?

The syndrome of Calcinosis, Raynaud's phenomenon, Esophageal dysfunction, Sclerodactyly and Telangiectasias is classified within the subset of limited scleroderma [1]. Nail fold capillaroscopy with a pattern different than that seen in systemic sclerosis can help in the diagnosis of limited scleroderma. In limited scleroderma, while the nailfold capillaries are dilated, there usually are no drop out areas devoid of capillary loops as there typically are in diffuse systemic sclerosis.

Table 1. Cardinal Clinical Manifestations of Systemic Sclerosis

- Antecedent Raynaud's phenomenon
- Skin thickening of the hands, arms, legs, as well as the face – the buccal aperture is narrowed – neck and trunk
- Involvement of the lungs, heart, gastrointestinal tract and/or kidneys
- Presence of antinuclear antibodies.

What is the ten-year prognosis of limited and diffuse scleroderma?

Diffuse (systemic) scleroderma generally has a worse prognosis, with a 40 to 60% survival at ten years, as opposed to a > 70% survival at ten years for limited scleroderma [1]. The most frequent causes of death in systemic sclerosis are: renal - hypertension, hazard ratio (HR) = 1.9; cardiac, HR = 2.8; and pulmonary, HR = 1.6. The presence of anti-topoisomerase I antibodies imparts a HR of death of 1.3 [5].

What is the typical course of limited scleroderma?

Most patients with limited scleroderma have Raynaud's phenomenon for years before other signs of organ involvement are seen. These patients are less likely to develop severe heart or kidney disease than those with diffuse scleroderma. However, pulmonary arterial hypertension, biliary cirrhosis, small intestinal malabsorption, and large artery occlusive disease with resultant digital ischemia and amputations are the most serious manifestations of limited scleroderma [1].

What is the pathogenesis of systemic sclerosis?

Stimulation of fibroblasts with excessive synthesis of type I and type III collagen and other connective tissue matrix proteins, with accumulation in the skin and other organs, underlies the pathogenic mechanism of systemic sclerosis. Stimulation of fibroblasts is caused by a variety of cytokines including transforming growth factor-beta, epidermal growth factor, endothelin [6] platelet derived growth factor and tumor necrosis factor beta.

Endothelial cell damage by cytokines also contributes to the pathogenesis with resultant edema, increased vascular permeability and release of von Willebrand's factor. Platelet activation along with mononuclear cell products results in further damage to the vascular endothelium. Reduced oxygen delivery to tissues progresses to ischemia, necrosis and eventual fibrosis. Serum autoantibodies are present in 95% of patients with systemic sclerosis, although their role in pathogenesis is uncertain.

An interesting possibility in the pathogenesis of systemic sclerosis is *micro-chimerism*. Chimerism is the presence of more than one genotype in an organism. Micro-chimerism is the presence of cells from another individual at low levels. Women with systemic sclerosis and who have been pregnant have increased fetal cells in their skin, circulation and spleen compared with women without systemic sclerosis who have been pregnant [7]. In this vein, Graft versus host disease has several of the features of systemic sclerosis.

Which autoantibodies are associated with scleroderma?

The most common autoantibody associated with **limited scleroderma** targets the kinetochore portion of the centromere, anti-centromere antibodies, and occurs in 45 to 70% of patients. In **diffuse scleroderma**, antibodies to topoisomerase I (anti-Scl-70) occur in approximately 35% of patients. Anti-topoisomerase I antibodies are also associated with pulmonary interstitial

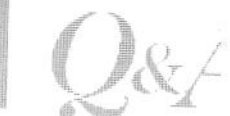

fibrosis. Although not very sensitive, these autoantibodies are very specific: anti-centromere for limited scleroderma and anti-topoisomerase I for diffuse scleroderma.

What is scleroderma renal crisis?

In the past, renal disease was a major cause of mortality in systemic sclerosis. The scleroderma renal crisis usually occurs in patients with diffuse disease and typically occurs in the setting of rapid worsening of diffuse cutaneous involvement. The rapid onset of severe arterial hypertension, microscopic hematuria, and proteinuria progresses to overt renal failure. Occasionally a crisis can occur without hypertension. There is an association between the scleroderma renal crisis and antibodies to RNA polymerase III antigen. Since the advent of angiotensin-converting enzyme (ACE) inhibitors, survival among patients with this complication has greatly improved if treatment is started promptly [(8)]. Currently, pulmonary interstitial fibrosis is the leading cause of death in diffuse SSC.

How is systemic sclerosis treated?

Treatment is still vexing. The most widely used drug in the treatment of systemic sclerosis had been D-penicillamine. This drug acts as an immunomodulator and interferes with collagen cross-linking. A large retrospective study showed improvement in skin thickening after two years and improved five-year survival compared to untreated patients [(9)]. However, it is unclear if D-penicillamine is truly effective in SSc, and many authorities now advocate abandoning its use in this disease. Cyclophosphamide, methotrexate and cyclosporine A have shown promising results in several small studies. A recently published, double-blind, randomized, placebo-controlled trial of cyclophosphamide for interstitial lung disease in systemic sclerosis showed modest improvement, but at considerable toxicity [(10)]. Chlorambucil, 5- fluorouracil, aspirin and dipyridamole have been shown to be ineffective [(1)].

KEY POINTS

- Systemic sclerosis (SSc) is a connective tissue disease characterized by overproduction of collagen and subsequent sclerosis of skin and internal organs.
- Raynaud's phenomenon occurs in the large majority of patients and can precede the other manifestation by months or years.
- Variants include limited scleroderma, or the CREST syndrome, and localized scleroderma, such as morphea.
- Treatment is still suboptimal and evolving.
- Angiotensin converting enzyme inhibitors have significantly improved the prognosis for patients with the scleroderma renal crisis. Long-acting nifedipine is beneficial for Raynaud's phenomenon.

CHAPTER 13

MIXED CONNECTIVE TISSUE DISEASE

Edward P Cutolo

What is the Mixed Connective Tissue Disease?

Mixed connective tissue disease (MCTD) manifests overlapping features of systemic lupus erythematosus (SLE), polymyositis and systemic sclerosis (SSc)[1].

What clinical manifestations are associated with mixed connective tissue disease?

Common symptoms include Raynaud's phenomenon and diffusely swollen fingers and hands. Systemic lupus erythematosus - associated findings include polyarthritis, lymphadenopathy, facial erythema, pericarditis, pleuritis, leukopenia and thrombocytopenia. Polymyositis - associated findings include Raynaud's phenomenon, proximal muscle weakness, elevated serum levels of creatine kinase and a myopathic pattern on electromyogram[2]. Systemic sclerosis - associated findings include tight skin, pulmonary fibrosis and hypomotility or dilatation of the esophagus.

Which autoantibody is most commonly associated with the mixed connective tissue disease?

The most common autoantibody associated with MCTD is anti-ribonuclear protein antibody (RNP antibody), directed at the uridine rich small nuclear ribonucleoprotein (U1 snRNP)[3]. Of possible importance, Mairesse et al demonstrated very high titers of autoantibodies to the 73-KD heat shock protein in MCTD. These high titers were specific for MCTD, and were not seen in SLE, polymyositis or systemic sclerosis[4].

Which clinical feature is associated with a poor prognosis?

Pulmonary hypertension is the major factor contributing to either serious morbidity or mortality. The duration of disease prior to death in patients with pulmonary hypertension ranges from three to eleven years. Pulmonary hypertension occurs in up to 23% of patients[3].

Are there any serologic markers associated with the development of pulmonary hypertension in Mixed Connective Tissue Disease?

The presence of IgG anti-cardiolipin antibodies correlates with pulmonary hypertension-related deaths. Surprisingly, these patients did not have thromboembolic phenomenon or other features of the anti-phospholipid syndrome [(3)].

Is MCTD really a distinct clinical entity?

This point remains controversial among rheumatologists. However, the serologic markers, immunogenic association with HLA-DR4/HLA-DR2, and the clinical configuration of Raynaud's phenomenon, arthralgia, arthritis, diffusely swollen hands, myositis, esophageal motility disorders, and pulmonary impairment, support the distinction from other discrete connective tissue diseases [(3)].

How often are the kidneys involved in MCTD?

Approximately 25 percent of patients with mixed connective tissue disease will have renal involvement. Membranous glomerulonephritis is the most commonly associated nephropathy, and although usually mild, can progress to the nephrotic syndrome. Possibly due to the reno-protective role of anti-U1 RNP antibodies, diffuse proliferative glomerulonephritis is unusual. Malignant renovascular hypertension, such as occurs with systemic sclerosis, can also occur in MCTD.

How is mixed connective tissue disease treated?

Most patients with mild cases can be treated successfully with NSAIDs, or corticosteroids with cyclophosphamide, in severe cases [(3)].

KEY POINTS

- The mixed connective tissue disease (MCTD) is characterized clinically by features of systemic lupus erythematosus, polymyositis, and systemic sclerosis (scleroderma). Features of rheumatoid arthritis are sometimes seen as well.
- MCTD is characterized serologically by antinuclear antibodies in a speckled fluorescent staining pattern and by antibodies to ribonucleoprotein, anti-RNP antibodies, in very high titers.
- Treatment depends on organ involvement, and nonsteroidal antiinflammatory drugs alone suffice in mild disease.
- Corticosteroids at a dose of 1 mg/kg per day are required in more severe disease.
- Most of these patients have a better prognosis than patients who have one of the constituent diseases alone, although, there are exceptions.

CHAPTER 14

GIANT CELL ARTERITIS (TEMPORAL ARTERITIS, CRANIAL ARTERITIS) AND POLYMYALGIA RHEUMATICA

Edward P Cutolo

What is Giant Cell Arteritis?

Giant cell arteritis, also known as temporal arteritis or cranial arteritis because it commonly affects the external cranial arteries, is a systemic vasculitis that affects both medium and large arteries. It occurs in patients over 50-years-old, with the highest susceptibility in women and those of Northern European origin [1]. In fact, there is a striking difference in incidence and prevalence of giant cell arteritis and polymyalgia rheumatica by ethnicity. Scandinavians have the highest; blacks and Hispanic people, the lowest rates. An annual incidence of biopsy-proven giant cell arteritis in the population 50 years or more is 18 per 100,000 in Scandinavia and the United States. A five-year study by Salvarani, *et al.*, in Reggio Emilia, Italy revealed an annual incidence of giant cell arteritis of 8.8 per 100,000 persons over 50 years of age. One study conducted in Israel by Friedman, et al., showed the lowest recorded incidence of polymyalgia rheumatica, 0.5 per 100,000 [2,3].

What is the relationship of polymyalgia rheumatica to giant cell arteritis?

Polymyalgia rheumatica is also a syndrome affecting the elderly and is closely associated with giant cell arteritis, given the fact that half of the patients with giant cell arteritis have or had polymyalgia rheumatica. In addition, 10 to 15% of patients with polymyalgia rheumatica without symptoms of giant cell arteritis have this vasculitis on biopsy [1].

What is the pathogenesis of giant cell arteritis and polymyalgia rheumatica?

The pathogenesis of these two disorders is not fully understood; they may represent the same disease at different points of evolution. Inflammation of the arterial wall seems to be the result of a targeted immune response. While, inflammatory changes can extend to all layers of the blood vessel, the most severe changes occur in the intima, which becomes thickened, and in the inner media, which has the highest proportion of leukocytic infiltration. Biopsied arteries in pure polymyalgia rheumatica do not reveal arteritis. Newer research techniques have shown that cytokine mRNA derived from both lymphocytes and macrophages was found in temporal artery biopsy specimens from polymyalgia rheumatica as well as giant cell arteritis. Arteries from polymyalgia rheumatica did not show interferon gamma, however, which suggests that progression from the "subclinical vasculitis" of PMR to the overt vasculitis of giant cell arteritis may be mediated by this cytokine. Higher concentrations of interleukin-2 mRNA in the temporal arteries of patients with giant cell arteritis are associated with concurrent polymyalgia rheumatica [4, 5].

What are the clinical manifestations of giant cell arteritis?

Systemic symptoms include malaise, fatigue, fever, weight loss, night sweats and depression. The fever may be as high as 40° C (104° F) and giant cell arteritis can present as a fever of unknown origin. Pain and stiffness in the neck, shoulders and buttocks, as in polymyalgia rheumatica, may also appear. Manifestations related to arterial involvement include headaches and tenderness of the scalp especially over the temporal or occipital arteries. The temporal arteries may be erythematous and thickened. Aching or tiredness in the muscles on the involved side of the face, brought on by chewing and relieved by rest, is known as jaw or masticatory claudication. This symptom represents involvement of the maxillary artery and occurs in about half the patients with giant cell arteritis. It is nearly pathognomonic although masticatory claudication can occur in amyloidosis too. Pain felt behind the ear may be associated with vertigo and deafness.

Involvement of the aorta and other major vessels occurs in approximately 15% of patients and may result in aneurysm formation, dissection, stenosis, reduced blood pressure in one or both arms, and arm claudication [6, 7]. In fact, aortic aneurysm may be a delayed sequela of GCA, occurring years after GCA has remitted. On the average, thoracic aortic aneurysm develops ten years after giant-cell arteritis is diagnosed. However, aortic dissection and upper extremity large-artery stenosis can develop much sooner. Thoracic aortic aneurysm occurs about 17 times more frequently and abdominal aortic aneurysm about twice as frequently in patients with giant-cell arteritis as in the general population. Consequences of major artery involvement are stroke, upper extremity claudication, unequal upper extremity blood pressures, and bruits over the carotids, subclavian, and brachial arteries. An aortic regurgitation murmur can signify aortic involvement. Involvement of the coronary arteries can lead to myocardial infarction. Keeping in mind these complications of giant cell arteritis can allow earlier detection and decreased mortality[8].

Blindness, one of the most feared consequences of giant cell arteritis, occurs in about 10% of patients with untreated giant-cell arteritis, and is a result of ischemic optic neuritis[9] from involvement of the posterior ciliary or central retinal arteries. On funduscopic examination, a pale optic disc is characteristic.

How is polymyalgia rheumatica distinguished from polymyositis?

Polymyalgia rheumatica is typically associated with pain and severe morning stiffness in the neck, shoulders, buttocks, and thighs, whereas polymyositis is typically associated with proximal muscle weakness, less often with myalgia. As opposed to polymyositis, muscle strength is normal in PMR[10].There may appear to be muscle weakness, as patients may not exert themselves fully because of the pain. Muscle enzymes are normal in polymyalgia rheumatica.

When should giant cell arteritis be suspected?

Giant cell arteritis should be suspected in a patient +50 years old who has new onset headache, jaw claudication, fever and/or symptoms of polymyalgia rheumatica. Physical examination may yield thickened, tender or erythematous areas over the temporal artery, arterial bruits, asymmetric peripheral pulses and blood pressures, and the diastolic murmur of aortic regurgitation[11] (Figure 1).

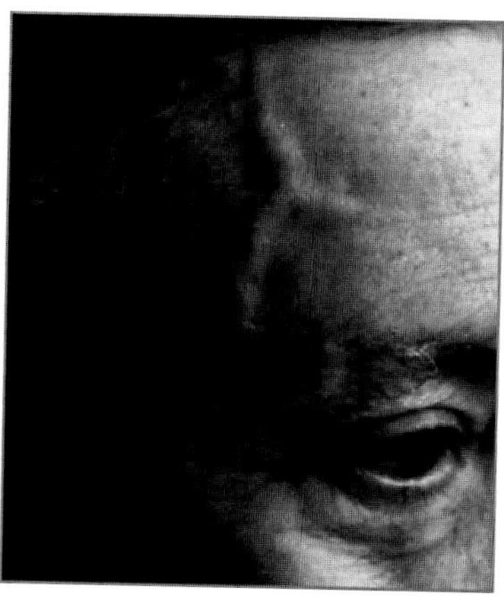

Figure 1. *Giant cell arteritis of the temporal artery. Enlarged right temporal artery. The artery can be thickened, tender and pulseless, although not invariably.*
Grassi, W, University of Ancona, Italy

What about the laboratory in GCA and PMR?

The cardinal laboratory findings are an erythrocyte sedimentation rate (ESR) greater than 50 mm per hour in 80% of patients with giant cell arteritis and greater than 40 mm per hour in 80% of patients with PMR, and an elevated C reactive protein, demonstrated in 100% of patients with biopsy proven giant cell arteritis in one study[12]. The C-reactive protein is generally greater than 8 mg/dL in giant cell arteritis or polymyalgia rheumatica. The use of both tests improves sensitivity. Elevations of these nonspecific markers of inflammation are very helpful in making the diagnosis of giant cell arteritis, although normal values do not exclude the diagnosis[12]. Up to 20% of patients with giant cell arteritis or PMR have a sedimentation rate < 40 mm per hour. Anemia of chronic disease is a concomitant of GCA/PMR. In fact, anemia falsely elevates the ESR, making C-reactive protein the acute phase reactant of choice, particularly when there is anemia. An increased alkaline phosphatase of liver origin occurs in one-third to one half of patients with both polymyalgia rheumatica and giant cell arteritis. Interestingly, the white blood cell count is normal in GCA and PMR, unless glucocorticoids are being used.

What establishes the diagnosis of giant cell arteritis?

The gold standard in establishing the diagnosis of giant cell arteritis is a biopsy of the temporal artery. To decrease the risk of false negative biopsy results due to "skip" lesions, a three to six cm section of artery should be obtained and the pathologist should do a serial sectioning of the specimen. A negative biopsy on one side should prompt consideration of a biopsy on the other temporal artery[6]. However, even in the most experienced hands, there is a false negative biopsy rate of about 10%, and the diagnosis must be made clinically, by signs, symptoms and response to glucocorticoids.

When should glucocorticoid treatment be started relative to the temporal artery biopsy?

Due to the serious nature of this disease, with the risk of blindness, stroke or myocardial infarction, appropriate treatment with a glucocorticoid should not be delayed while awaiting biopsy and diagnostic confirmation. Biopsy findings remain positive seven to fourteen days after initiation of medical treatment[13] when alteration in the histopathology occurs.

What other diagnoses should be considered?

Entities that may mimic giant cell arteritis include dental conditions, trigeminal neuralgia, sinus disease, otological conditions, retinal vascular accident, Wegener's granulomatosis, polyarteritis nodosa, Takayasu's arteritis and occasionally amyloidosis. Of note, vasculitides other than GCA can involve the temporal artery. The differential diagnosis of polymyalgia rheumatica includes rheumatoid arthritis, hypothyroidism, neoplastic disease, cervical spondylosis, multiple myeloma, leukemia, osteomyelitis and miliary tuberculosis [14].

What is the treatment of polymyalgia rheumatica and how does it differ from giant cell arteritis?

Polymyalgia rheumatica is treated with prednisone, 10 to 15 mg a day. Responses are often dramatic, with relief within 48 to 72 hours [10]. Giant cell arteritis is treated with prednisone, 0.7 to 1 mg/kg a day, usually in the range of 60 mg a day. Recent data suggest the importance of aspirin in the treatment of giant cell arteritis. In one recent study, the use of aspirin in a dose of 100 mg a day, in addition to a glucocorticoid, was associated with a reduced risk of visual loss and stroke compared to patients treated with a glucocorticoid only. Cranial ischemic complications, e.g., blindness and/or stroke, developed in 13% of the patients treated with prednisone only, and in 3% of the aspirin plus steroid-treated patients ($P = 0.02$) [15]. The mechanism of aspirin's effect probably is inhibition of interferon gamma, which functions in the pathogenesis of arterial damage in giant cell arteritis and which is not suppressed by glucocorticoids.

In GCA, a glucocorticoid, e.g., prednisone or prednisolone, is used at a daily dose of 0.7 – 1 mg/kg for about a month or six weeks, when symptom control and return to normal of the acute phase reactants is usually achieved. Then, the glucocorticoid is tapered by 10% of the daily dose at two to three weekly intervals. A rebound in the ESR is not an indication for increasing the dose of glucocorticoid, unless there is a recrudescence of symptoms. A return to the previous higher dose is usually effective in such situations. A regimen for treating patients with impending blindness or stroke includes aspirin, half of a 325 mg tablet, and a very high dose of methylprednisolone intravenously, 1gm a day for the first 72 hours, followed by aspirin, half of a 325 mg tablet, and oral prednisone, 0.7-1 mg/kg a day. This very high dose corticosteroid treatment has not been studied in randomized controlled trials.

The myriad side effects of glucocorticoids are a strong impetus to keep an end-point of treatment in mind and to taper the dose as soon as is feasible, as discussed above. Practically every patient on a glucocorticoid for three months or longer should be on supplemental calcium, 1500 mg day, and vitamin D, 400 – 800 units a day, and if there is osteoporosis on DEXA scanning, a bisphosphonate unless contraindicated. The American College of Rheumatology has published guidelines on preventing or treating glucocorticoid-induced osteoporosis[16]. Patients with giant cell arteritis and PMR are most likely to relapse during the initial 18 months of treatment and within one year of withdrawal of steroids. After two years, between one-third and one-half of patients can stop steroids.

KEY POINTS – GIANT CELL ARTERITIS

- Giant cell arteritis (GCA) is a vasculitis of large and medium size arteries.
- It often involves the temporal arteries, and occurs in people 50 years of age and over.
- Headache is a common symptom of GCA. The headache can be of any type, and can be intermittent or steady.
- A feared complication is blindness. Stroke and myocardial infarction are other possible complications.
- GCA can present as fever of unknown origin.
- The Westergren erythrosedimentation rate is usually, but not invariably, 50 mm per hour or higher.
- Lately, the C-reactive protein is being used more for its greater sensitivity than the erythrosedimentation rate.
- A person suspected of having GCA should be biopsied as soon as possible. A symptomatic artery, such as the temporal or occipital artery, should be biopsied.
- Glucocorticoids are imperative as soon as the diagnosis is suspected. Prednisone or prednisolone is started at an initial dose of 0.7 - 1mg/kg, usually 40-60 mg a day, in three divided doses if the patient appears ill. The biopsy will not be obscured by glucocorticoid treatment for one or two weeks.

- Response is usually dramatic and corticosteroids can be tapered slowly.
- A late complication of GCA, important to keep in mind, is aortic aneurysm, which can occur several years later when the cranial arteritis is ostensibly spent.

KEY POINTS – POLYMYALGIA RHEUMATICA

- Polymyalgia rheumatica (PMR) is a painful condition of the shoulder and hip girdle muscles.
- The neck and low back can be involved, and patients complain of severe morning stiffness.
- This condition also occurs in individuals 50 years of age or over.
- Fifteen percent of patients with PMR have GCA. Conversely, 50% of patients with GCA have PMR.
- The Westergren erythrosedimentation rate is usually, but not invariably, 40 mm or higher in the first hour. As in giant cell arteritis, the quantitative C-reactive protein assay adds much to diagnostic accuracy.
- It is not necessary to do a temporal artery biopsy in a patient with PMR who does not have symptoms or signs of GCA, although it is important to follow closely for the development of GCA.
- Corticosteroids are dramatically effective in PMR. Complete relief of pain characteristically occurs within a week, and this point can be used as a diagnostic feature.
- Lower doses of a glucocorticoid than for GCA are used: 10-15 mg daily initially and tapered as symptoms permit.

CHAPTER 15

OTHER VASCULITIDES

Keith S Kanik

What is vasculitis?

Vasculitis is inflammation of the walls of blood vessels. The vasculitides, as a group, are not rare [1], and vasculitis can occur in arteries as large as the aorta, or in microscopic vessels such as arterioles, capillaries or venules. Although generally an autoimmune process, vasculitis also can be infectious in etiology. Conditions mimicking vasculitis are nutritional deficiencies such as scurvy, and thrombotic disorders such as the antiphospholipid antibody syndrome, Buerger disease (thromboangiitis obliterans), cholesterol emboli, and atrial myxoma.

Early signs of vasculitis are nonspecific and include fever, fatigue, weight loss and poor appetite. Organ ischemia distal to vessel inflammatory occlusion is a common pathophysiologic pathway of signs and symptoms (Figure 1). Laboratory abnormalities common to most forms of vasculitis include anemia, thrombocytosis, and elevated inflammatory indices such as the erythrocyte sedimentation rate (ESR) and C-reactive protein. Although an elevated ESR is not diagnostic, ESRs over 100 mm per hour are suspicious for a vasculitis.

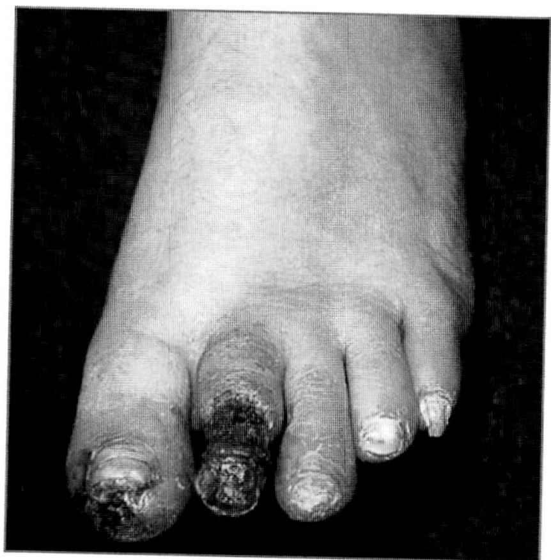

Figure 1. *This patient has developed gangrene of his toes consequent to systemic necrotizing vasculitis of medium-sized blood vessels. Taggart, A, Mussgrave Park Hospital, Belfast, Northern Ireland.*

Likewise, a C-reactive protein greater than 10 mg/dl is suggestive of systemic vasculitis in the absence of an acute infection

What are the different types of vasculitis?

There are many different types of vasculitis, and classification systems are based on size of the vessel, organ system affected, and whether another connective tissue disease is associated (Table 1 and Table 2). Examples of systemic vasculitis are Wegener's granulomatosis, Takayasu's arteritis, giant cell arteritis, Churg Strauss vasculitis, polyarteritis nodosa, microscopic polyangiitis, and Henoch Schönlein purpura. Other forms of vasculitis include those associated with Behçet's syndrome, systemic lupus erythematosus, Sjögren's syndrome and rheumatoid arthritis[2]. Drug induced vasculitis can result from various medications, such as penicillin, sulfonamides, phenytoin, allopurinol, and propylthiouracil. The latter has been incriminated in a Wegener–like syndrome.

There are various classification schemes for the vasculitides; one of the most commonly used is by size of the vessels involved (Table One).

Table 1. Classification of Selected Vasculitides by Size of Vessel Involved

Small Vessel Vasculitis (vessels without muscular walls, i.e., arterioles, capillaries, and venules)

Cutaneus leukocytoclastic vasculitis (Leukocytoclasia is the presence of nuclear debris around the damaged vessels.)

Henoch Schonlein purpura

Cryoglobulinemic vasculitis

Vasculitis that is part of a another connective tissue disease, such as, rheumatoid arthritis, systemic lupus erythematosus, Sjogren's syndrome)

Wegener's granulomatosus

Churg-Strauss syndrome

Microscopic polyangiitis

Medium-sized Vessel Vasculitis (including small arteries with muscle in the vessel wall)

Polyarteritis nodosa

Large vessel vasculitis (the aorta and its major branches)

Takayasu

Giant cell (temporal) arteritis

Table 2. Typical Clinical Manifestations of the Vasculitides by Size of Vessel Involved

Small Vessel, Cutaneous leukocytoclastic Vasculitis (formerly, hypersensitivity vasculitis)

Palpable purpura

Urticaria

Occasionally, glomerulonephritis or GI involvement

Small Vessel, Systemic Vasculitis

Skin and vital organ involvement

Medium-sixed Vessel Vasculitis

Skin ulcers

Livedo reticularis

Gangrene of the fingers and toes

Mononeuritis multiplex

Vital organ vasculitis

Large Vessel Vasculitis

Bruit over large arteries

Asymmetric blood pressures

Intermittent claudication and limb ischemia

Aortic dissection and aneurysm

Blindness, stroke

Are different vasculitides more common in different regions and populations?

Wegener's granulomatosis is more common in higher latitudes, and microscopic polyangiitis in lower latitudes. Takayasu's arteritis is most common in Asia and in young women. Giant cell arteritis is most common in the elderly and those with Scandinavian backgrounds. Henoch Schonlein related vasculitis is most common in children, Behçet's syndrome in those of middle eastern and Asian backgrounds [3].

How is vasculitis diagnosed?

The gold standard is a biopsy, although this procedure is not always available. Angiographic findings of multiple aneurysms, tapered narrowings and irregularities suggest vasculitis but are not definitive. Atherosclerotic changes, vasospasm and cocaine abuse can all cause similar angiographic alteration. The resolution of magnetic resonance angiography is generally not sufficient for diagnosis and should not be used as a foundation for diagnosis.

What is Wegener granulomatosis?

This vasculitis is a granulomatous inflammatory process of the small and medium-sized vessels, most commonly affecting the upper respiratory system, lungs, kidneys, eyes, and ears. However, many other organ systems can be involved. In the lungs there are diffuse pulmonary infiltrates (Figures 2, 3), lymphadenopathy, pulmonary hemorrhage, and occasionally even overlap with

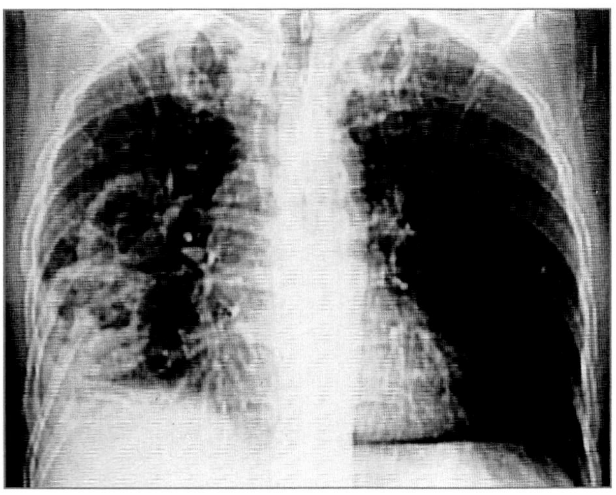

Figure 2. *Wegener Granulomatosus. A chest X-ray with several nodules in evidence, some with cavitation.*

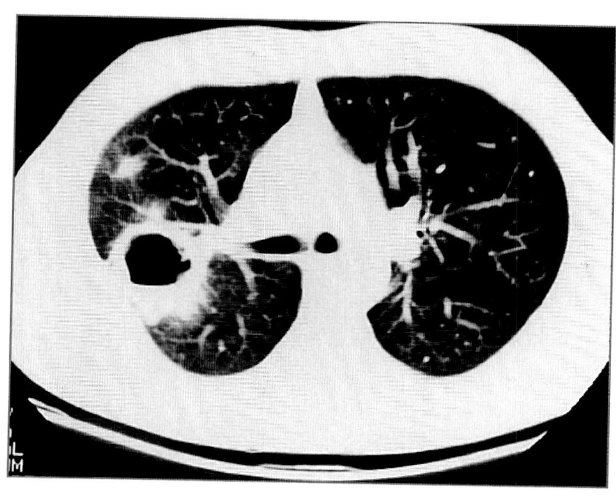

Figure 3. CT scan of the chest showing cavitary lesions in the right lung in a patient with Wegener granulomatosis.

giant cell arteritis [4]. Diagnosis is made on the basis of a biopsy showing necrotizing granulomatous vasculitis. Diagnosis may be aided by the presence of an autoantibody, cytoplasmic antineutrophil cytoplasmic antibody, or cANCA. Like other autoantibodies, cANCA per se does not diagnose Wegener granulomatosis. However, in conjunction with other clinical factors, it supports the diagnosis and is useful for monitoring therapy [5]. The antigen to which cANCA forms is a serine protease called proteinase-3.

What is Churg-Strauss syndrome?

Also known as allergic granulomatosis and angiitis, this vasculitis is very rare. It occurs in about 2.4 people per million. Churg-Strauss syndrome is a vasculitis of small- and medium-sized vessels. It is associated with asthma and the presence of eosinophilia in the blood. Organs affected are the lungs, skin, viscera, nerves, and kidneys. Diagnosis is based on biopsy showing eosinophilic infiltrates, angiitis, and extramural necrotizing microgranulomas [6]. Churg-Strauss syndrome is associated with the perinuclear antineutrophil cytoplasmic antibody, pANCA, whose antigen is myeloperoxidase.

What is polyarteritis nodosa?

This small and medium-sized vessel vasculitis affects the skin, nerves, kidneys, viscera, and testes. Arteritis of the vasa nervorum of the radial nerve causes a characteristic wrist drop, a downwardly flexed wrist with the inability to dorsiflex. A similar problem can involve the foot – foot drop. One can hear such a patient coming as the foot slaps the ground. The lungs are typically spared in polyarteritis. Diagnosis of this systemic necrotizing vasculitis is based on biopsy or less accurately, on angiogram [6]. The latter shows microaneurysms, suggestive, but not entirely sensitive or specific. Hepatitis B infection causes polyarteritis in about 40% of cases.

What is microscopic polyangiitis?

This vasculitis affects arterioles, capillaries or venules. It can occur in multiple organ systems including the lungs and kidneys as glomerulonephritis and pulmonary capillaritis with pulmonary hemorrhage, and it is most commonly associated with the presence of pANCA [6], with myeloperoxidase the antigen.

What is Cryoglobulinemic Vasculitis?

This form of vasculitis is caused by immune complexes that have the physical property of precipitating in cool temperatures. Mixed cryoglobulinemia, composed of complexes of IgM with rheumatoid factor activity against IgG, is caused by hepatitis C infection in at least 80% of cases. A small and medium-sized vessel vasculitis occurs when the complexes deposit in the vessel wall and

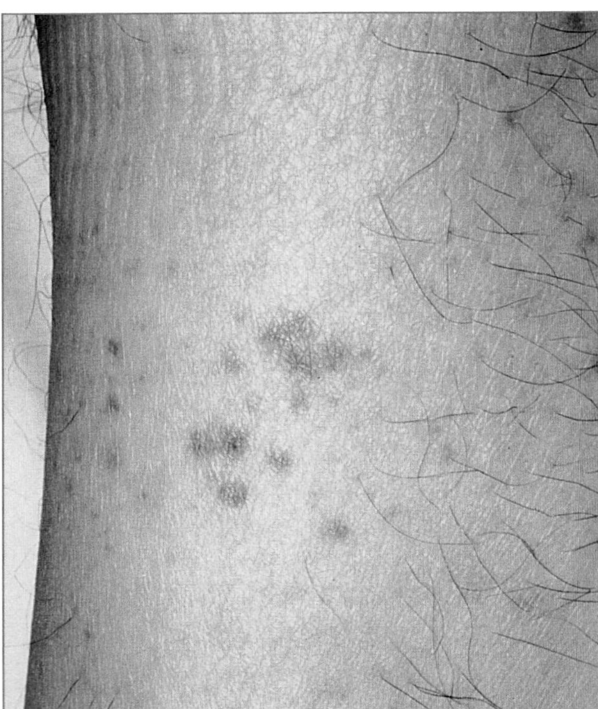

Figure 4. *Palpable purpura in this patient with small vessel vasculitis.*

activate complement. Serum rheumatoid factor is positive, and serum levels of C4 are depressed more than C3 in this disease. Cryoglobulins are detected by bringing the patient's serum sample to the lab at body temperature, or there can be loss of immune complexes by precipitation, then the centrifugation at body temperature of the serum, and then refrigeration of the serum at 4 degrees C for at least 72 hours. The cryoprecipitate can then be characterized as to its constituents. HCV RNA is concentrated in the cryoprecipitate.

Clinically, cryoglobulinemic vasculitis manifests as cutaneous *palpable purpura* of the legs from leukocytoclastic vasculitis (Figure 4), glomerulonephritis, arthralgias, fatigue, and neuropathy. Palpable purpura is an expression of small vessel vasculitis involving the arterioles, capillaries and venules. It is not specific for cryoglobulinemic vasculitis [7]. The term leukocytoclasia connotes the presence of much nuclear debris on biopsy microscopy and characterizes small vessel vasculitis. Meltzer's triad is palpable purpura, arthralgias and fatigue from cryoglobulinemia. Mesenteric and CNS vasculitis occur uncommonly. Raynaud's phenomenon and livedo reticularis can accompany the vasculitis.

Therapy of severe life-threatening disease consists of treating the immune-inflammation with glucocorticoids and cyclophosphamide. Plasmapheresis can be helpful. If present, treating the hepatitis C infection with pegylated interferon-alpha alone or combined with ribavirin is indicated.

See the Clinical Laboratory in Rheumatology chapter for more information about cryoglobulinemia.

How is vasculitis treated? (Table 3)

The treatment of choice for any life-threatening vasculitis is the combination of a corticosteroid and daily oral cyclophosphamide [8]. Milder forms of the disease may respond to a corticosteroid alone, or less toxic therapies such as monthly pulse cyclophosphamide, oral weekly methotrexate or oral azathioprine [9]. There are case reports of biological therapies being used for treatment of a diverse group of vasculitides [10]. Infliximab in particular has been used in both giant cell arteritis and Behçet's syndrome (see below), which supports the need for future study in this area. In Takayasu arteritis, surgical grafting plays an important role in the management of these patients. In Wegener's granulomatosus, management of subglottic stenosis with nonsurgical techniques and the outcome of tracheostomy for life-threatening tracheal involvement are discussed in a recent article [11].

Table 3. Generalities of Treatment of the Vasculitides

Observation may suffice in mild cases of cutaneous vasculitis

Where relevant, discontinue the offending medication

Treatment with a glucocorticoid and cyclophosphamide are often necessary in cases of systemic vasculitis (e.g., PAN, MPA, Wegener's) with vital organ involvement (e.g., kidney, heart, lungs, GI). Methotrexate can be helpful in maintaining remission after cyclophosphamide

Refer to a rheumatologist for recalcitrant or life-threatening cases

Constant reassessment is necessary to evaluate for a flare of vasculitis. One method is by the VITAL assessment tool.

(Bacon PA, Moots RJ, Exley A. VITAL (Vasculitis Integrated Assessment Log) assessment of vasculitis. Clin Exp Rheumatol 1995;13:275-8.)

KEY POINTS

- The consequences of the vasculitides are from ischemia distal to vessel luminal narrowing from inflammation.
- The most common vasculitis is small vessel vasculitis, often caused by a hypersensitivity reaction to medication.
- Clinical manifestations suggestive of vasculitis are palpable purpura, abdominal pain, bloody stools, hematuria, hypertension, and neuropathy, especially mononeuritis multiplex with wrist drop or foot drop.
- The anti-neutrophile cytoplasmic antibody (ANCA) test has become an important part of the workup of vasculitis.
- Cytoplasmic anti-neutrophil cytoplasmic antibodies, cANCA, are associated primarily with Wegener granulomatosis and crescentic, necrotizing glomerulonephritis. The antigen of cANCA is proteinase-3.

- Perinuclear anti-neutrophile cytoplasmic antibodies, pANCA, are associated primarily with microscopic polyangiitis and the Churg-Strauss syndrome (allergic granulomatosis and angiitis), The antigen of pANCA in these vasculitic diseases is myeloperoxidase.
- There is some overlap in disease specificity; that is, some patients with Wegener's granulomatosis will be pANCA positive and some patients with microscopic polyangiitis will be cANCA positive.
- The hepatitis C virus causes most cases of mixed cryoglobulinemia. The hepatitis B virus causes a large percentage of cases of polyarteritis nodosa.
- The treatment for vasculitis depends on the organ involved and the acuity of disease progression.
- The small vessel vasculitis associated with medication, often responds to discontinuation of the medication.
- Alternatively, in small vessel vasculitis or the other vasculitides, if there is vital organ involvement, such as mesenteric arteritis, coronary arteritis, renal involvement, or involvement of the central nervous system, a corticosteroid is necessary. For life-threatening cases, cyclophosphamide can be life saving.

CHAPTER 16

RELAPSING POLYCHONDRITIS

Rajani P Shah

What is relapsing polychondritis?

Relapsing polychondritis is a syndrome characterized by widespread, intermittent but progressive inflammation and destruction of cartilaginous structures and other connective tissue. It is believed to be an autoimmune disorder of unknown etiology in which antibodies to type II collagen are present [(1)]. All types of cartilage may be involved, including the elastic cartilage of the ears and nose, the hyaline cartilage of the peripheral joints, the fibrocartilage at axial sites, and the cartilage in the tracheobronchial tree [(1)].

What systems are mostly affected by the disease?

The most common manifestation occurs in the auricular area, which heralds more widespread involvement. There is pain, erythema and warmth involving the cartilaginous structure of the ear. The earlobes are spared due to their lack of cartilage. When there is inflammation of the entire external ear, infection is the cause. Continued and repetitive inflammation can lead to external auditory canal narrowing and deafness. The auricle can become misshapen, with a forward floppy appearance, often referred to as cauliflower ear.

Other manifestations of relapsing polychondritis include polyarthritis, seen in about half of patients. There is usually an asymmetric, migratory, nonerosive arthritis [(2)]. Scleritis and episcleritis are also common. Life threatening involvement of the respiratory tract can occur. Tracheal involvement can lead to difficulty breathing, stricture, stridor, and the need for emergency intervention. If the nasal septum is involved, a saddle nose deformity may develop. Another serious complication involves the cardiovascular system. Patients can develop aortic aneurysm and acute aortic insufficiency, as well as other valvular abnormalities and complete heart block [(3)]. Patients frequently have systemic complaints of fatigue, fever and weight loss.

Who is affected by relapsing polychondritis?

Men and women are affected with equal frequency. The disease can occur in the young and elderly, with the most likely onset between the fifth and sixth decade. It primarily affects Caucasians but occurs in other ethnic groups as well [4].

How is the diagnosis of relapsing polychondritis made?

The diagnosis is made by clinical presentation. The sedimentation rate is usually elevated, but this test is non-specific. A biopsy of inflamed cartilage is helpful, but it is not necessary except in ambiguous cases [4]. Relapsing polychondritis is often difficult to diagnose early in its course; in a series of 66 patients, the mean delay from the time medical attention was sought for symptom onset until diagnosis was 2.9 years [4].

Are there any specific markers that would be helpful in making the diagnosis?

There are no specific laboratory data that assist with the diagnosis. The clinical findings are sufficient to make the diagnosis in most patients.

What is the treatment available for relapsing polychondritis?

The first line of therapy for mild disease is a nonsteroidal anti-inflammatory drug. If the symptoms are more severe, a corticosteroid with or without an immunosuppressive drug is indicated.

Can relapsing polychondritis occur with other diseases?

Yes. Some of these associated diseases are systemic vasculitis, rheumatoid arthritis, systemic lupus erythematosus, Sjögren syndrome, inflammatory bowel disease, myelodysplastic syndromes, and Hodgkin disease. **M**ucosal and **G**enital **U**lcers with **I**nflamed **C**artilage constitute the MAGIC syndrome, an overlap of relapsing polychondritis with Behçet's syndrome [2].

What is the prognosis for relapsing polychondritis?

In most patients, relapsing polychondritis is a progressive disease. A 1986 series showed the overall survival rate at five years was 74% and at ten years was 55% [5]. The most common cause of death was pneumonia [5].

KEY POINTS

- Relapsing polychondritis is an inflammatory disease involving destruction of cartilaginous and connective tissues.
- Onset is usually in the fifth or sixth decade.
- The diagnosis is clinical; biopsy is not necessary. There are no specific markers that assist in making the diagnosis.
- Treatment for mild disease is an NSAID. More severe manifestations require corticosteroids and immunosuppressive drugs.
- Overall survival rate at five years is 74% and at ten years is 55%.

CHAPTER 17

BEHÇET'S SYNDROME

Bryan A Bognar

How is Behçet's syndrome diagnosed?

There is no specific laboratory test for Behçet's syndrome. As such, it remains a clinical diagnosis. The International Study Group for Behçet's syndrome proposed the following criteria for diagnosing Behçet's syndrome [1]:

- Relapsing oral ulcers, including major and minor aphthous or herpetiform ulcers, occurring at least three times in one year (Figure 1);

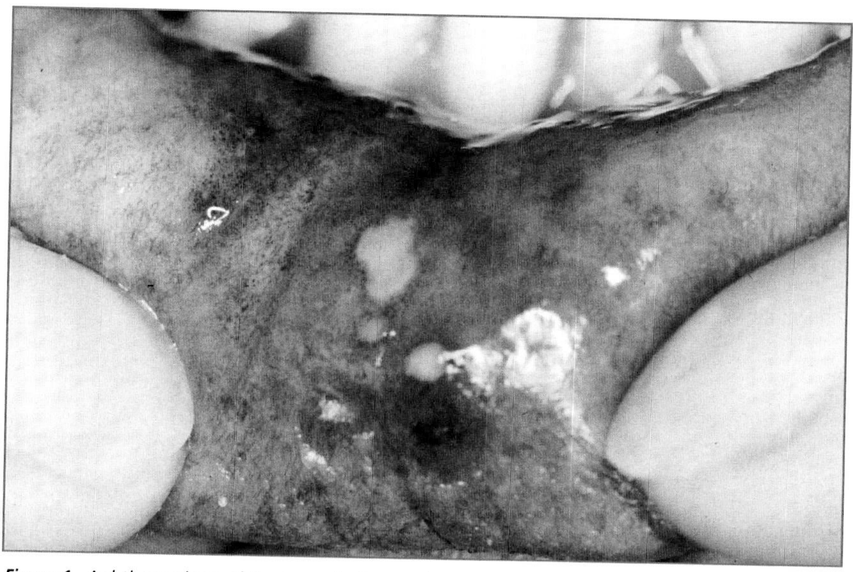

Figure 1. Aphthous ulcers of the lower lip in a patient with Behçet syndrome. These ulcers are painful and can occur anywhere in the mouth.

In addition, patients must have at least two of the following:

- Recurrent genital ulcers;
- Inflammatory eye lesions, including anterior or posterior uveitis, or cells in the vitreous on slit lamp examination;

- Skin lesions, including erythema nodosum, pseudofolliculitis, papulopustular lesions, or acneiform nodules in postadolescent patients not on corticosteroids;
- Positive skin pathergy test (see below) (Figure 2).

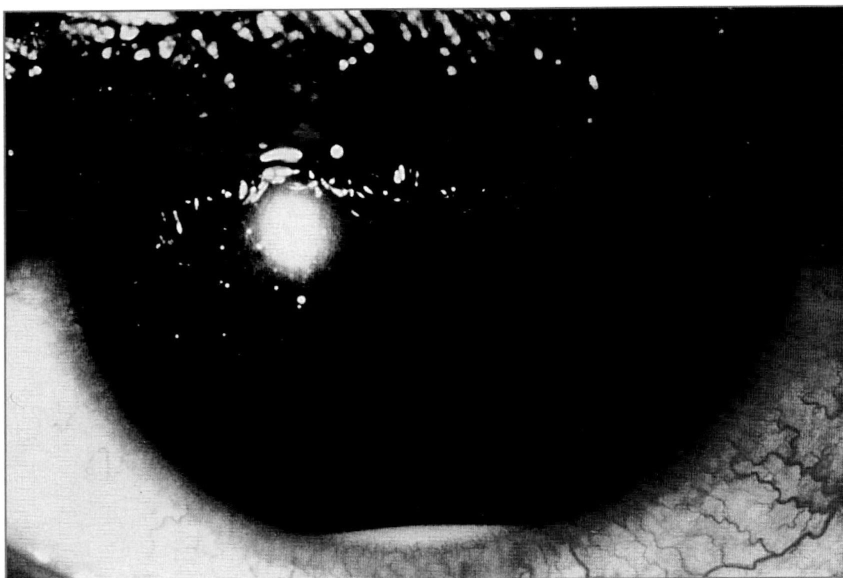

Figure 2. Hypopyon iritis in Behçet's syndrome. Note the cells in the anterior chamber at 6:00, sometimes visible without a slit lamp.

Who was Behçet?

Hulusi Behçet was a Turkish dermatologist who, in 1937, first recognized the triad of recurrent ocular inflammation and aphthous oral and genital ulcers as a distinct clinical entity [(2)].

Who gets Behçet's syndrome?

While men and women appear equally susceptible to Behçet's syndrome, the frequency of more severe disease is higher in men. The age of most patients at diagnosis ranges from 15 to 45 years. Ethnically, people from the Mediterranean Basin, the Middle East (especially Turkey with a prevalence of 80 to 370 per 100,000 people), and Japan have the highest prevalence of Behçet's syndrome. In England and the United States, prevalence figures range from 12 to 64 persons per million [(3)].

What causes Behçet's syndrome?

The etiology of Behçet's syndrome is unknown. The pathogenesis probably involves autoimmunity to some degree. The major histocompatibility complex HLA-B51 probably plays a role in pathogenesis in this syndrome. Pathologically, vasculitis of the vasa vasorum is the major site of involvement in the large vessel component of Behçet's syndrome [4].

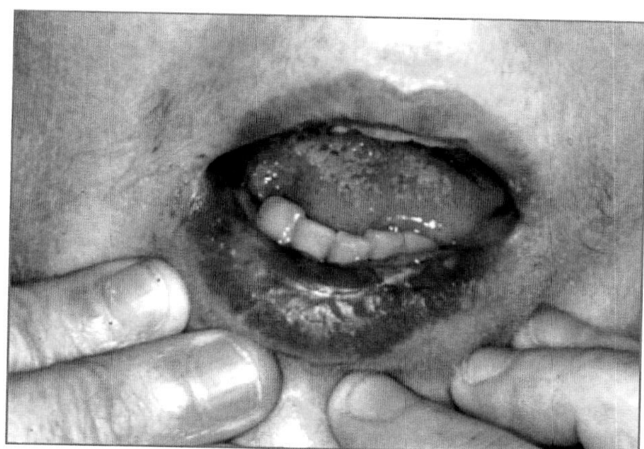

Figure 3. *Behçet syndrome. The oral lesions are a sine qua non of Behçet syndrome and are painful, aphthous ulcers that recur at least three times a year. They can appear anywhere on the oral mucosa and are usually the first manifestation of Behçet syndrome.*

Taggart A, Musgrave Park Hospital, Belfast, Northern Ireland.

What are the Clinical Manifestations of Behçet's Syndrome?

The most common clinical features of Behçet's syndrome include recurrent oral ulcers (nearly 100%) (Figure 3), recurrent genital ulcers (nearly 80%), skin lesions (approximately 75%), eye lesions (approximately 66%), and skin pathergy (variable) [3]. Skin pathergy is the formation of a sterile pustule after sterile pin prick. Hypopyon iritis, pus in the anterior chamber of the eye, although unusual these days, is very suggestive of Behçet's syndrome.

What are some of the other less common but serious clinical manifestations of Behçet's syndrome?

Other important clinical features of Behçet's syndrome are:

- Neurologic manifestations, including headache, cerebellar and pyramidal signs, sensory deficits, papilledema, cranial nerve palsies, and meningoencephalitis;
- Vascular manifestations, including superficial thrombophlebitis, vasculitis, arterial aneurysms, and occlusions of major veins or arteries;

- Arthritis, including nonerosive, monoarticular and oligoarticular involvement of the knees, ankles, wrists, and elbows;
- Gastrointestinal manifestations, including ulcerative lesions from the mouth to the anus, often confused with Crohn's disease.

What are the clinical characteristics of the oral aphthous ulcers seen in Behçet's syndrome?

The aphthous ulcers of Behçet's syndrome can occur anywhere in the oral cavity, including the gingiva, lips, buccal mucosa, and tongue. Aphthous ulcers are described as minor (<1 cm) or major (>1 cm), and they almost always occur in crops. They typically have sharply demarcated erythematous borders with a grayish pseudomembrane. Aphthous ulcers take one to three weeks to heal, and it is uncommon for them to scar.

How is Behçet's syndrome treated?

Treatment of Behçet's syndrome is determined by the clinical manifestation being targeted [3]. For example, aphthous ulcers initially can be treated with a topical corticosteroid, tetracycline solution, or topical sucralfate. For more severe or refractory ulcers, systemic prednisone, methotrexate or levamisole have been used. Immunosuppressive agents such as cyclosporin, azathioprine or cyclophosphamide are typically reserved for the most serious or potentially life-threatening complications of Behçet's syndrome, such as sight –threatening ocular disease, neurologic manifestations or arteritis. Clinical trials of anti-tumor necrosis factor-alpha agents for Behçet's syndrome are underway [5].

KEY POINTS

- Behçet syndrome is diagnosed clinically; there is no specific laboratory test.
- The most common clinical features are recurrent, painful oral ulcers, recurrent genital ulcers, eye inflammation, and skin lesions including pathergy.
- The "classic" oral ulcer of Behçet syndrome is a painful aphthous ulcer characterized by sharply demarcated erythematous borders with a grayish pseudomembrane.

- This syndrome may be accompanied by a number of potentially serious manifestations, including neurologic, vascular, and gastrointestinal complications.
- Treatment of Behçet syndrome ranges from topical corticosteroids for aphthous ulcers to systemic immunosuppressives for more severe manifestations

CHAPTER 18

THE (SERONEGATIVE) SPONDYLOARTHRITIDES

Bryan A Bognar

What is meant by the term "seronegative" and "spondyloarthritis?"

A feature common to all of the seronegative spondyloarthropathies (SpA) is a negative rheumatoid factor and antinuclear antibody test, hence the term "seronegative." The term spondyloarthritis connotes inflammation of the joints of the vertebral column as well as the peripheral joints[1].

What clinical entities fall under the rubric of (seronegative) spondyloarthritis?

Ankylosing spondylitis, the prototype, enteropathic spondyloarthritis, including ulcerative colitis and Crohn's disease, reactive arthritis (ReA), psoriatic arthritis, and juvenile spondyloarthritis primarily make up the spondyloarthritides[1]. Some authors would include Behçet's syndrome, and the so-called SAPHO syndrome (see below) because of occasional sacroiliac joint involvement.

Why do we group these seemingly disparate syndromes together?

In each case, the etiology or pathogenesis is poorly understood. There is clearly a genetic component; however, genetics are neither necessary nor sufficient to completely explain the pathogenesis of this group of arthropathies. Linking clinical features include a tendency toward sacroiliitis and characteristic extra-articular manifestations, such as mucocutaneous, ocular or cardiac involvement[1].

What is the association between the genetic human leukocyte antigen (HLA) system on chromosome 6 and the spondyloarthritides?

There is a strong association with HLA-B27[2]. At least 23 different subtypes of HLA-B27, designated B*2701 to B*2723 have now been identified. B*2705 is by far the most frequent subtype found in Caucasians, and it is highly associated with ankylosing spondylitis. Exceptions to the susceptibility to ankylosing spondylitis conferred by some HLA B27 subtypes are seen among the Western African population of Senegal and Gambia. The risk of developing ankylosing spondylitis in these HLA B27 positive individuals is lower than in HLA B27 positive Caucasians, and HLA B27 subtypes do not seem to explain this finding. There is posited a non-HLA B27 protective factor reducing the susceptibility to ankylosing spondylitis in this population.

B*2704 is also a frequent subtype and is the predominant subtype associated with the spondyloarthritides in Chinese and Japanese patients.

The fascinating question is what is the biological significance of this link?

Whether the pathogenesis of the spondyloarthritides is directly related to the HLA system is still being studied. Several mechanisms by which HLA-B27 molecules could operate to increase susceptibility to these diseases have been proposed, yet none has been proven. One prominent theory is the unfolded protein response (UPR): HLA B27 is a very large macromolecule that slowly unfolds in the endoplasmic reticulum (ER). This macromolecule can get "stuck" in the ER exposing arthitogenic epitopes to immune-active cells. Comparison of HLA-B27 molecules that are and are not associated with spondyloarthritides have shown that if HLA-B27 induces arthritis by presenting peptides to CD8+ T cells, the ability to present peptides terminating in tyrosine is critical.

What about the frequencies of HLA-B27, and the relative risks of ankylosing spondylitis or reactive arthritis, in patients with HLA-B27?

The association of HLA-B27 with the spondyloarthritides represents one of the strongest hereditary markers of disease[2]. Over 90% of Caucasoids with ankylosing spondylitis are HLA-B27 positive, whereas the frequency of this antigen in Caucasoids without ankylosing spondylitis is about 6%. A person born with a certain type of HLA-B27 antigen has an 87 times risk of ankylosing spondylitis compared to a patient without that HLA-B27 antigen. As discussed, there are several different types of HLA-B27 molecules. There are at least seven subtypes of HLA-B27 antigen that are associated with ankylosing spondylitis[3]. HLA-B27 positive relatives of patients with ankylosing spondylitis have a higher rate of this disease than HLA-B27 positive individuals without such a family history.

Furthermore, there is a considerable difference in ankylosing spondylitis rates in HLA-B27 positive people from different parts of the world. HLA-B27 subtype 03 occurs frequently in Africans, but it is not associated with ankylosing spondylitis. This observation probably explains why ankylosing spondylitis is uncommon among African Americans with the HLA-B27 antigen [(4)]. The HLA-B27 subtypes 02, 04, 05 and 06 are more strongly associated with this condition. About 30 to 50% of Caucasoids with reactive arthritis are HLA-B27 positive. The relative risk of a Caucasoid who is HLA-B27 positive and is exposed to one of the etiologic agents of reactive arthritis is 37 compared with someone who is HLA-B27 negative.

What features help distinguish between inflammatory back pain and mechanical back pain?

The inflammatory back pain of the spondyloarthritides is typically worse in the morning and abates somewhat as the day goes on, and there is significant morning stiffness of the back. In ankylosing spondylitis, back pain begins before age 40, and it is insidious in onset [(1)]. The presence of inflammatory bowel disease, reactive arthritis, or psoriasis should heighten one's suspicion of a spondyloarthritis. It should be mentioned that the peripheral arthritis of inflammatory bowel diseases parallels the activity of the bowel disease, but the spondylitis is independent of bowel disease activity. On the other hand, mechanical back pain gets worse as the day goes on, there is little morning stiffness, and onset can be at any age. Mechanical back pain is usually acute in onset.

What are the signs and symptoms of ankylosing spondylitis?

Ankylosing spondylitis, the prototype spondyloarthritis, is a chronic inflammatory disease of the spine and peripheral joints. There is predilection for the sacroiliac joints, characterized by back pain and progressive stiffness, worse in the morning. Ankylosing spondylitis characteristically affects young male Caucasoids, with a peak age of onset between 20 and 30 years of age. The prevalence of ankylosing spondylitis in white European and North American populations is between one in 100 and one in 250 in men. The male to female ratio is about five to one, and the disease is rare in Black people, most likely a result of different HLA alleles. As the disease progresses, there can eventuate a fixed, stooped posture with loss of lumbar lordosis and ankylosis of the SI joints (Figures 1, 2). Peripheral arthritis, particularly of the hips, shoulders and knees, occurs in up to 50 percent of patients and chronic changes occur in 25 percent. In addition, the eyes, heart, and lungs can be affected in ankylosing spondylitis. Acute iritis, aortic regurgitation, and upper lobe fibrocavitary disease are examples of such involvement. Other complications of ankylosing spondylitis are IgA nephropathy and amyloidosis.

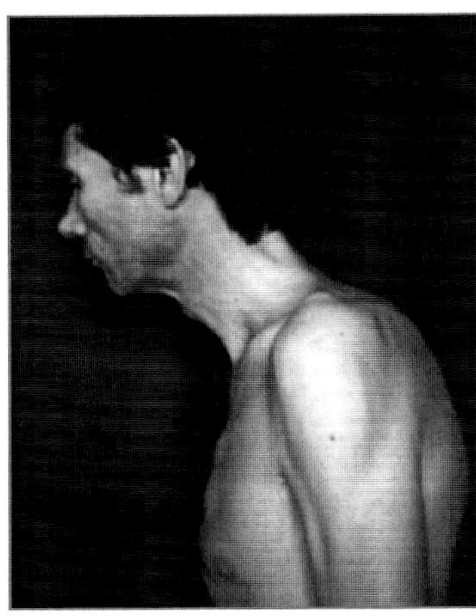

Figure 1. *This young man demonstrates the fixed, stooped posture of late ankylosing spondylitis.*

Grassi W, University of Ancona, Italy.

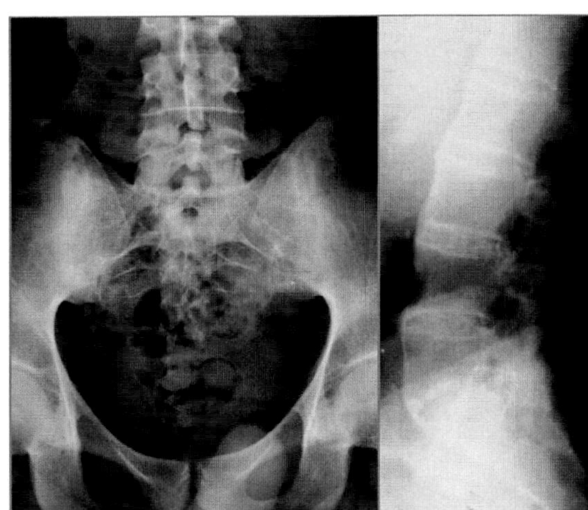

Figure 2. *Left panel: There is bilaterally symmetrical, complete ankylosis of the sacroiliac joints. No sacroiliac joint space is visible.*

Cimmino MA, Garlaschi G, Silvestri E. Univerisyt of Genova ,Italy.

Right panel: lateral view of the lumbosacral spine. Thin, marginal syndesmophytes are noted, bridging the intervertebral disc spaces. The syndesmophytes are formed from calcification of the annulus fibrosis.

Tagnocco A, Valesini G, Rome University, "La Sapienza", Italy.

What is reactive Arthritis, and which microorganism can cause it?

The term reactive arthritis (ReA) was at first meant to denote that the arthritis was not a direct result of viable microorganisms invading the joint, but rather a result of an infection at a distance to the joint. An immune mechanism was set in motion to microbial antigens reaching the joints. Recently elucidated exceptions are *Chlamydia trachomatis* and *Chlamidophila pneumoniae (formerly, Chlamydia pneumoniae)*. These organisms are found live in the joint. Reactive arthritis can be postvenereal, or endemic, or postdysenteric, or epidemic. The postvenereal form is caused by *Chlamydia trachomatis* or *ureaplasma urealyticum*. Postdysenteric reactive arthritis can be caused by salmonella, shigella, campylobacter species, or yersinia. If an individual is born with a particular type of HLA-B27, and he is exposed to one of these microbes, there is about a 20% chance of contracting reactive arthritis. Overall, 5% of people exposed to a specific infection develop reactive arthritis. If the individual has the HLA B27 antigen, there is approximately a 20% chance. Post streptococcal arthritis in adults, perhaps a forme fruste of acute rheumatic fever sparing the heart, is another form of reactive arthritis, though without sacroiliitis/spondylitis or an HLA B27 association. Poncet disease is a reactive arthritis to infection elsewhere by Mycobacteria spp.

The articular manifestations of reactive arthritis are most typically a pauci- or oligoarticular (four or less peripheral joints) or monoarticular antritis, often involving the large joints of the lower extremities with large effusions. Sacroiliitis and spondylitis with syndesmophytes (boney bridges emanating from the lateral vertebral margins or bodies) occur in at least 20% of patients.

Extraarticular manifestations of ReA include *urethritis* , *conjunctivitis, acute anterior uveitis, oral sores, keratoderma blennorrhagicum* - palmar and plantar lesions resembling pustular psoriasis, *circinate balanitis* – a circular rash on the

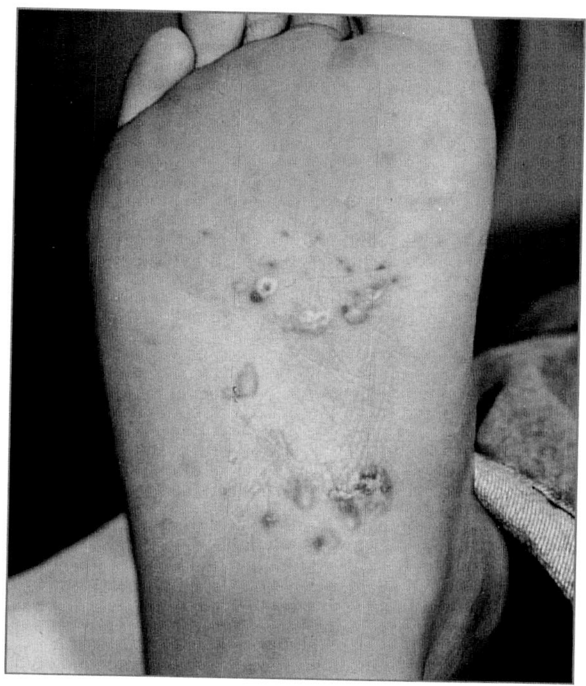

Figure 3. *This patient with reactive arthritis has keratoderma blennorrhagicum on the soles of his feet. These lesions are indistinguishable from those of pustular psoriasis, another example of the cross-over of some of the features of the spondyloarthritides.*

glans penis, and *heel pain* – a manifestation of **enthesitis** (see below), sometimes facetiously referred to as "lover's heel." Patients with post dysentery ReA can have urethritis, and patients with post-venereal ReA can have diarrhea. ReA can also be associated with HIV disease.

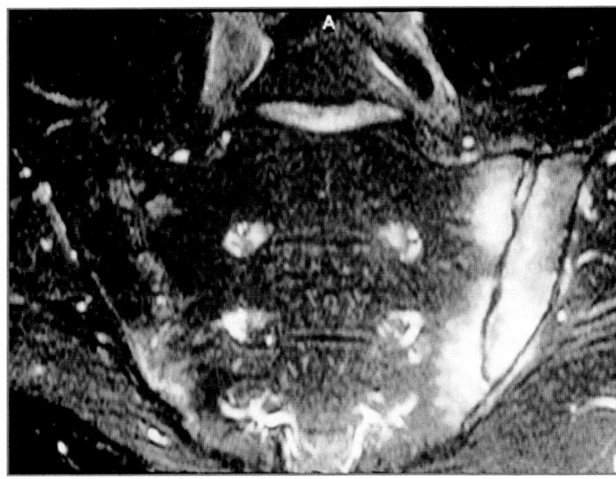

Figure 4. *A T_2 weighted fat suppressed MRI of the sacroiliiac joints. The asymmetric involvement is consistent with a diagnosis of psoriatic spondyloarthropathy or reactive spondyloarthropathy.*

What are the signs and symptoms of psoriatic arthritis?

The prevalence of psoriatic arthritis is approximately 0.1 percent of the population in the United States and United Kingdom. Psoriasis affects about 1% of the general population, and psoriatic arthritis affects up to 25% of individuals with psoriasis. There are several patterns of psoriatic arthritis. Distal interphalangeal joint arthritis of the fingers is considered the most specific for psoriatic arthritis, but it is not the most common pattern. The most frequent

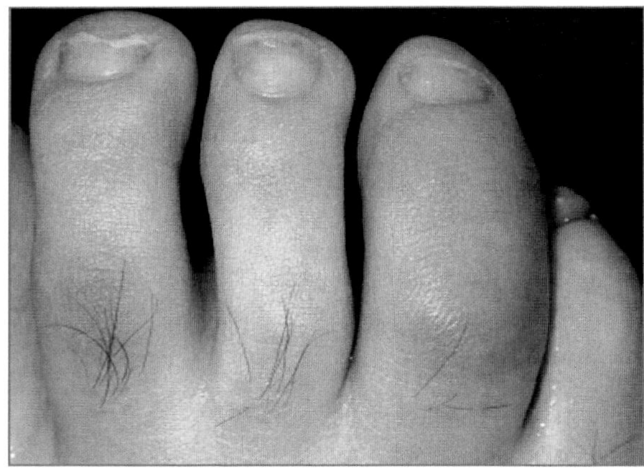

Figure 5. *Psoriatic arthritis. Note the diffusely inflamed fourth toe (sausage digit) and dystrophic nails -- important clues to psoriatic arthritis.*

Filippucci E, Grassi W, University of Ancona, Italy.

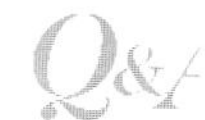

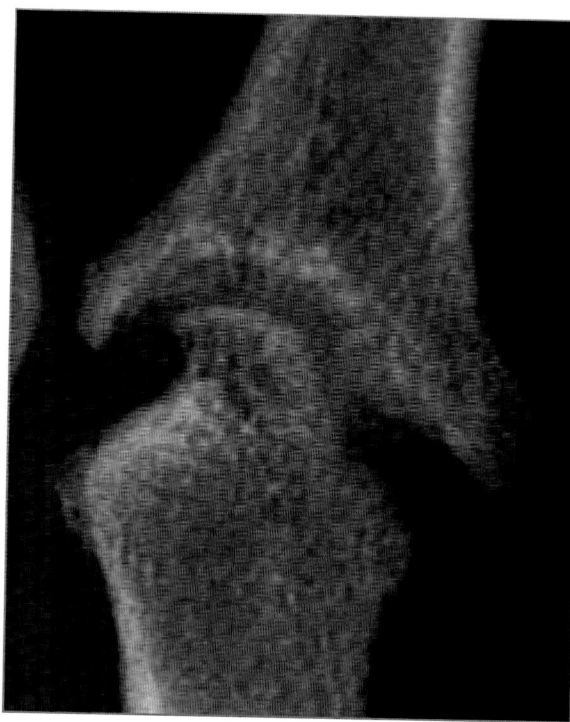

Figure 6. *This X-ray of a finger of a patient with psoriatic arthritis shows a characteristic, though not invariable, sign, the so-called pencil-in-cup deformity.*

Grassi W, Filippucci E, University of Ancona, Italy

presentations are *polyarthritis*, involvement of five or more peripheral joints, followed by oligoarthritis or pauciarticular arthritis, involvement of less than five peripheral joints. Distal involvement alone occurs in less than 20 percent of cases. The spondyloarthropathy is usually found in association with peripheral joint involvement, but can occur alone. Sacroiliac involvement in psoriatic and reactive spondyloarthropathy can be unilateral or asymmetrical, as well as bilaterally symmetrical (Figure 4). On the other hand, sacroiliac involvement in the other two main spondyloarthropathies, ankylosing spondylitis and the

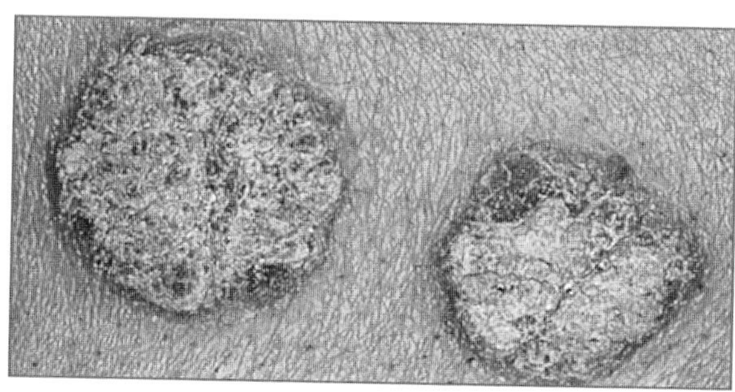

Figure 7. *Psoriasis. The silver scales are typical of psoriasis. If a scale is lifted with a sterile needle, there are punctate bleeding sites underneath. This sign is called the Auspitz phenomenon.*

Doria, A, Rondinone R, University of Padova, Italy.

spondyloarthropathy of the inflammatory bowel diseases, ulcerative colitis and Crohn's disease, is typically bilaterally symmetrical. Arthritis mutilans, which can occur with any of the patterns, is a particularly destructive arthritis with osteolysis (absorption) of phalanges and metacarpals and shortening of the fingers: telescoping of the digits called *main en lorgnette*, or opera glass hand [5]. Arthritis mutilans can occur in rheumatoid arthritis and the arthritis of multicentric reticulohistiocytosis as well.

In common with the other spondyloarthropathies, psoriatic arthritis is characterized by **enthesitis** – inflammation at the attachment of tendons or ligaments to bone. Sausage-shaped swelling of the digits – dactylitis – is also characteristic of psoriatic arthritis, as it is of reactive arthritis (Figure 5).

X-rays can show the pencil-in-cup configuration, with tapering of the proximal part of the joint and splaying of the distal part (Figure 6).
Skin disease usually precedes joint involvement by years, but in about 15%, arthritis precedes skin involvement. Moreover, the degree of skin involvement does not necessarily parallel that of joint involvement. It is important to look for psoriatic patches "hiding" in the umbilicus, under the hair of the scalp, in the intergluteal cleft, or on the perineum (Figure 7).

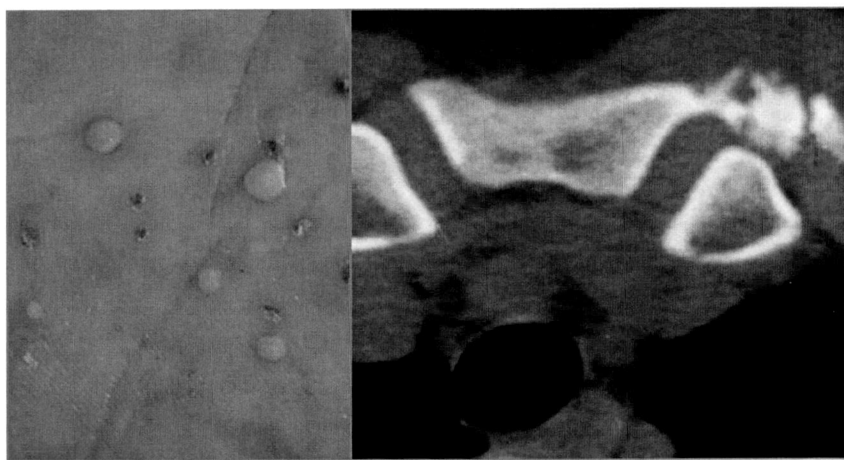

Figure 8. *Left panel: Palmar pustulosis in this patient with SAPHO.*
Grassi W, University of Ancona, Italy.

Right panel: Computed tomography shows hyperostotic and erosive lesions of the left first costochondral and chondrosternal junctions.
Trotta F, University of Ferrara, Italy and Santilli D, Parma Hospital, Italy.

Nail involvement might be the only dermatologic indication of psoriasis. There are several types of nail abnormality in psoriasis: Onycholysis - separation of the nail from the nail bed from subungual keratosis; multiple pitting; horizontal ridging; and oil drop discoloration – a brown-yellow staining. Interestingly, about 80 percent of patients with psoriatic arthritis, but 20 percent of patients with psoriasis without arthritis, have nail abnormalities. Severe cases of psoriatic arthritis are suggestive of concomitant HIV disease, and the latter should be excluded before treating these patients with methotrexate.

What is the SAPHO syndrome?

Sternocostoclavicular hyperostosis is also known as the SAPHO syndrome - an acronym unifying the clinical features of synovitis, acne, pustulosis, hyperostosis, and osteomyelitis (which is sterile). The SAPHO syndrome most prominently involves the anterior chest wall, and is associated with neutrophilic skin lesions, especially palmoplantar pustulosis and acne conglobata or acne fulminans (Figure 8)[6]. Clinical descriptions of this syndrome appear most often in the Japanese and European literature under a variety of names, including acne-associated spondyloarthropathy, chronic recurrent multifocal osteomyelitis, and pustulotic arthroosteitis. This syndrome is not associated with HLA-B27.

How are the spondyloarthritides best treated?

Aggressive physical therapy is of great importance in the management of the spondyloarthropathies[7]. Extension exercises and deep diaphragmatic breathing exercises are to be emphasized because the spondyloarthropathies tend to bring the patient into a flexed posture, and the costovertebral joints are involved, impairing this mechanism of breathing. Patients must stop smoking. The nonsteroidal anti-inflammatory drugs, especially indomethecin, are beneficial, but must be used with great care, if at all, if the patient has inflammatory bowel disease. Bowel perforation is a real risk. Sulfasalazine can be useful[8]. Methotrexate and gold are of use for the peripheral arthritis of psoriasis[9]. Treating Chlamydia trachomatis with a combination of a tetracycline product and rifampin for about three months might cure postvenereal reactive arthritis[10].

Treating the enteric pathogens does not shorten the course of postdysentery reactive arthritis. The tumor necrosis factor alpha blockers have recently been approved by the FDA for treatment of ankylosing spondylitis and psoriatic arthritis.

What is the prognosis of the spondyloarthritides?

Most patients can lead productive lives with proper management.

KEY POINTS

- The spondyloarthritides (SpAs) include ankylosing spondylitis, the enteropathic arthropathies (ulcerative colitis and Crohn disease), reactive arthritis, and psoriatic arthritis.
- There is a strong association between HLA-B27 and the SpAs, a fact that highlights the role of immunogenetics in these disorders.
- Each of the distinct SpAs is often associated with characteristic extra-articular mucocutaneous, ocular, or cardiac (e.g., aortic regurgitation) manifestations.
- Indomethacin tends to be the most effective NSAID for most of the SpAs although sulfasalazine is preferable for the enteropathic arthropathies.
- Recently, the tumor necrosis factor-alpha blockers have been added to the armamentarium against ankylosing spondylitis and psoriatic arthritis.

CHAPTER 19

SARCOID ARTHRITIS

Harold M Adelman

Sarcoidosis is a multisystem, T-cell driven disease of unknown etiology [1]. It is characterized by non-caseating granulomata that can involve any organ. The lung, skin, eye, liver, nervous system, and heart may be prominently involved in sarcoidosis [2]. Approximately one third of patients with sarcoidosis have musculoskeletal involvement [3]. There are two kinds of sarcoid arthritis [4, 5]. An acute, symmetrical arthritis with a predilection of the ankles and feet occurs. There may be marked periarticular inflammation. When this kind of sarcoid arthritis is associated with erythema nodosum and pulmonary hilar lymphadenopathy, it is called Lofgren's syndrome. Nonsteroidal antiinflammatory drugs usually suffice in treatment, although corticosteroids are sometimes necessary. Lofgren syndrome has an excellent prognosis, running its course in two to four months [4].

The second form of sarcoid arthritis is more destructive. This is a chronic arthritis with acute flares. The fingers may be diffusely swollen – sausage digits from sarcoid dactylitis (Figure 1). X-rays show distal osteolysis and cystic bony lesions.

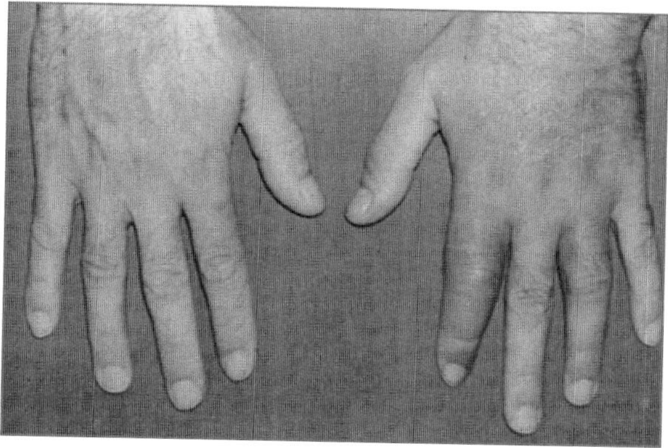

Figure 1. *This patient has sarcoid dactylitis of the left second finger. Notice the diffuse swelling of the digit because of wide-spread tendinitis. The left ring finger is involved to a lesser degree.*

Bell AI, Musgrave Park Hospital, Belfast, Northern Ireland.

In its most severe form, arthritis mutilans occurs with bony destruction and deformity of the fingers. Prednisone at a dose of 30 to 60 mg daily is usually required, and the arthritis tends to recur [5].

What joints are most often affected by gouty arthritis attacks?

Fifty percent of initial attacks occur in the first metatarsophalangeal joint (podagra). Ninety percent of patients with gouty arthritis will have involvement of this joint at some time during the course of their disease, although, almost any joint can be affected in gouty arthritis. The least affected is the hip joint, probably because of the relatively higher temperature in this joint [3]. Uric acid is more soluble at higher temperatures.

What are the risk factors for gouty arthritis?

Surgery may precipitate a gouty attack, which usually occurs several days after the operation [3]. Other risk factors include stress, trauma, alcohol use, starvation, infection and sudden changes in uric acid concentration, increased or decreased [3]. This latter fact accounts for the 20 to 30% of patients with an attack of gouty arthritis who have a normal serum uric acid level at the time of their attack. If uric acid levels are repeated over time, the patient eventually will be found to have hyperuricemia.

What about certain drugs that precipitate gouty attacks?

These drugs include cyclosporine, aspirin, loop and thiazide diuretics, pyrazinamide, niacin and hyperalimentation. In addition, the expectorant guaifenesin in cough syrups, and radio contrast dyes, by acutely lowering serum uric acid, can precipitate an attack in a predisposed individual.

Which foods precipitate gouty attacks?

Foods with high purine content, including meat, liver, beer (guanosine), spinach, mushrooms, peas, beans, asparagus, sardines, and anchovies acutely elevate serum uric acid [3].

What are the complications of untreated gout?

Tophi are deposits of solid monosodium urate in connective tissues (Figure 2). Gouty tophi tend to form at areas of friction, as is the case for rheumatoid nodules. Thus, there is a predilection for the olecranon process and the extensor surface of the forearm, and over the Achilles tendons. Occasionally, the monosodium urate drains though the skin, and has a toothpaste consistency. This characteristic is helpful diagnostically when present. Tophaceous gout generally arises after about ten years of untreated gout, but some postmenopausal women with osteoarthritis, especially if on diuretics, can develop tophi over their Heberden's nodes. This finding can occur even before having an attack of gouty arthritis. Untreated, tophi can progress to involve joints, renal, and even cardiac structures.

Joint X-rays sometimes show erosions with overhanging margins, unusual in other erosive arthropathies (Figure 2).

What is the best treatment for acute gouty attacks?

Non-steroidal anti-inflammatory drugs (NSAIDs) are the first-line medications. Aspirin is generally avoided due to the biphasic effect of salicylates on serum urate, resulting from renal uric acid retention at lower doses and uricosuria at high doses[4]. A glucocorticoid can be given by injection, intramuscular or intraarticular, if the patient is not able to take medication by mouth[4].
Oral prednisone, 20-40 mg a day for three or four days and then tapered over one to two weeks, is useful if an NSAID is contraindicated or has failed. ACTH, 40-80mg intramuscularly, followed by 40 mg every 6-12 hours for several days if necessary, is also effective and is preferred by some rheumatologists.

Most rheumatologists now feel that colchicine, the time-honored drug for acute gouty arthritis, should no longer be given in the acute setting because of its gastrointestinal side effects at high doses. Intravenous colchicine is very dangerous because of potential bone marrow toxicity[4] and should be avoided .

When should hospitalization be considered for a patient with an attack of gouty arthritis?

Patients are considered for hospitalization when oral therapy fails or patients are unable to take or tolerate oral medications. In addition, a patient with a

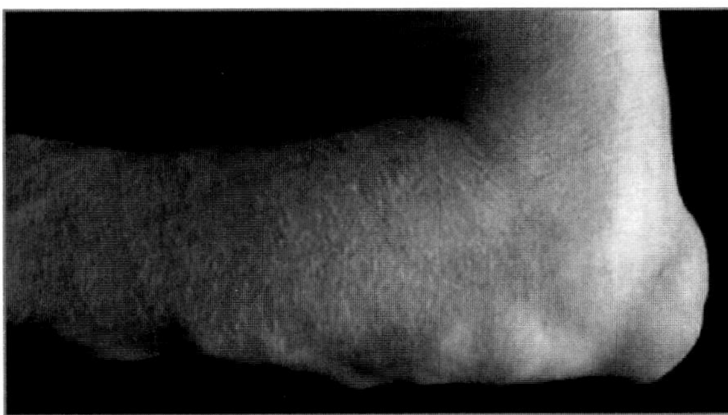

Figure 2. *Tophaceous gout. Tophi, in the olecranon bursa and over the extensor surface of the forearm of this patient with gout, are subcutaneous collections of monosodium urate crystals. They are usually an indication of chronic gout.*

Grassi, W University of Ancona, Italy.

first acute attack of acute arthritis in one joint should be hospitalized to rule out a septic joint.

Is there a role for treatment of asymptomatic hyperuricemia?

There are no data that prophylactic treatment of asymptomatic hyperuricemia provides benefit, except when the 24-hour urine uric acid excretion is > 800 mg [4].

Is obtaining a 24-hour urine for uric acid necessary when considering therapy?

A 24-hour urine for uric acid should be done, and over producers (>800 mg of uric acid in 24 hours) should be treated with allopurinol. Under excreters should be treated with allopurinol or uricosuric agents, such as probenecid if they have normal renal function and are not on aspirin, which counteracts probenecid [4].

When should the correction of hyperuricemia begin?

Indications for lowering serum uric acid include a history of two or three attacks of gouty arthritis, the presence of tophi, uric acid nephrolithiasis or a 24-hour urine uric acid excretion of > 800 mg. Agents to lower serum uric acid should

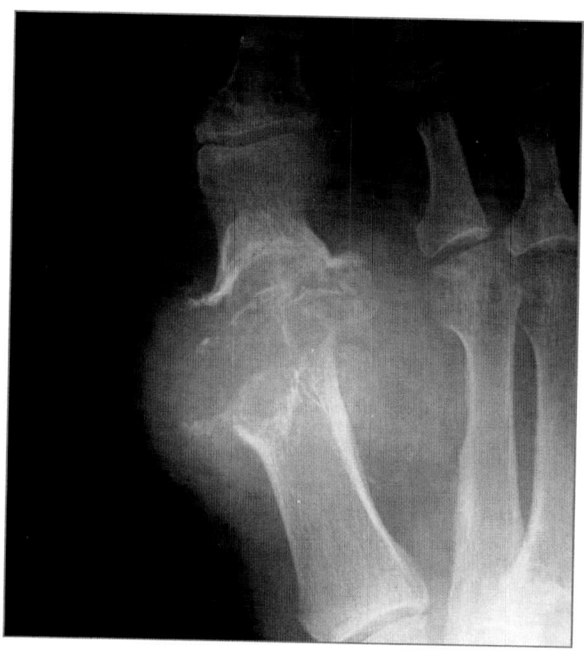

Figure 3. *This X-ray demonstrates the Martel sign: Notice the overhanging margin of the erosion caused by a contiguous tophus.*

Filippucci E, Grassi W, University of Ancona, Italy

begin about two weeks after all signs and symptoms of the acute attack have resolved, otherwise the attack might be prolonged by acutely lowering serum uric acid. Treatment is generally indefinite. Co-administration of colchicine is warranted to lessen the risk of breakthrough attacks of gouty arthritis. Colchicine can be stopped six months after the last attack of gouty arthritis.

What are the medications used for the treatment of chronic gout?

Colchicine prophylaxis, 0.6 mg twice daily, should begin about two weeks before treatment to reduce serum uric acid is initiated. The reason for this timing is to prevent breakthrough attacks of gouty arthritis as the serum uric acid is being reduced [(4)]. It is important to reduce the dose of maintenance colchicine if there is renal insufficiency; consequences of not doing so are myopathy and marrow suppression. In reducing uric acid, aim for a serum uric acid below 6 mg/dl, below 5 mg/dl if the patient has tophi. Allopurinol, a xanthine oxidase inhibitor, is effective for both over producers and under excreters of uric acid. The dose of allopurinol required to achieve the desired serum level of uric acid, below 6 mg/dl, is from 100 to 800 mg per day. Probenecid and sulfinpyrazone are effective uricosuric agents used in under excreters only.

The dose of allopurinol must be lowered if the creatinine clearance is reduced. Allopurinol can cause toxic epidermal necrolysis, especially in patients with reduced creatinine clearance. Other toxicities of allopurinol include vasculitis, granulomatous hepatitis, and a hypersensitivity reaction consisting of fever, rash, hepatitis, and eosinophilia. Allopurinol is not innocuous and must be used with care. Febuxostat is a new xanthine oxidase inhibitor for patients intolerant of allopurinol, and will be available in the near future.

KEY POINTS

- Gouty arthritis is an inflammatory condition caused by monosodium urate crystal deposition.
- Synovial fluid analysis demonstrates needle shaped, negatively birefringent crystals with a leukocyte count usually between 15,000-20,000.

- Factors that precipitate attacks are stress, trauma, surgery, alcohol use and sudden changes in uric acid concentration, up or down.
- Gout may lead to tophaceous (monosodium urate crystal) deposition in joints, subcutaneous tissues and renal parenchyma.
- The most effective treatment of acute gouty arthritis is an NSAID, or a corticosteroid for recalcitrant cases or if the patient cannot tolerate NSAIDs. High dose colchicine is not favored by many rheumatologists because of its GI side effects.
- Treatment of chronic gout usually is with allopurinol, with the goal of keeping the serum uric acid concentration less than 6.0 mg/dL, renal function permitting, and colchicine, 0.6 mg bid for six months after the last attack of gouty arthritis, to avoid a flare of gout while allopurinol is lowering the serum uric acid level.
- Do not start a uric acid lowering agent until two weeks after the acute attack has resolved.

PSEUDOGOUT – CALCIUM PYROPHOSPHATE DIHYDRATE (CPPD) CRYSTAL DEPOSITION DISEASE

What is CPPD crystal deposition disease?

It is a form of arthritis caused by deposition of CPPD crystals in the synovium and synovial fluid [1]. The acute form is referred to as pseudogout.

Are any other diseases associated with this entity?

Some metabolic diseases have been associated with CPPD, particularly hyperparathyroidism, seen in 7%. Other associations are hemochromatosis, hypothyroidism, amyloidosis, hypophosphatasia, and some electrolyte disturbances such as decreased magnesium and phosphate. This disorder has also been associated with trauma and occurs in the post-operative period, as does gouty arthritis. Granulocyte colony stimulating factor has also been associated with exacerbations of pseudogout in a case report; however, further studies are needed to establish this correlation [5].

Is there a familial pattern?

Some cases show an autosomal dominant pattern [6].

What is the pathogenesis of CPPD crystal deposition disease?

Crystals of CPPD in the synovial fluid are phagocytosed by polymorphonuclear leukocytes, which in turn release phlogistic mediators. In addition, studies of the synovial fluid have found high levels of inorganic phosphate. The inorganic phosphate, when in excess, can couple with other molecules and form CCPD crystals [6]. Sometimes, collections of CPPD crystals nested in the synovial membrane are "strip-mined" out by fluxes in synovial fluid phosphate concentrations.

How do patients usually present?

There are various clinical expressions of CPPD crystal deposition disease. The pseudogout form of CPPD crystal deposition disease, Type A, presents similarly to gout, with acute monoarticular and occasionally oligoarticular (four or less joints) pain and swelling. The knees, wrists and metacarpophalangeal joints are often affected. "The knee is to pseudogout what the first metatarsophalangeal joint is to gout." Symptoms, if untreated, can last two weeks or more. Patients can have a high fever and elevated white blood cell count. The average age of presentation is older than in gouty arthritis, and is about 72 years.

Other forms of CPPD crystal deposition disease are:

- **Type B** CPPD crystal deposition disease, or pseudorheumatoid arthritis. This variant is subacute and resembles rheumatoid arthritis in that it involves multiple joints. Synovianalysis with compensated polarized light and identification of the rhomboid-shaped, weakly positively birefringent crystals of calcium pyrophosphate dihydrate, will distinguish the process. Type B CPPD crystal deposition disease is rare, and represents 5% of the total of patients with this form of crystal arthritis.
- **Types C and D**, or **pseudo-osteoarthritis**. These variants look like osteoarthritis clinically. Type C manifests acute attacks of inflammation and detection of CPPD crystals in the joint fluid is telling. In type D, there are no acute attacks. Again, appropriate crystal identification on synovianalysis makes the diagnosis.

- **Type E** , or **lanthanic**, disease is the asymptomatic variant. There is chondrocalcinosis on X-ray, see below.
- **Type F** is the so-called **pseudoneuropathic** variant, and resembles Charcot arthropathy on X-ray.

Are there any suggestive radiologic findings?

The typical appearance is linear or punctate calcification in articular hyaline cartilage, and fluffy calcification in fibrocartilage (figure 4)[6]. This process is called chondrocalcinosis and represents the deposition of CPPD in cartilage. The prevalence of radiographic chondrocalcinosis is 15% in people 65-75 years of age, and up to 60% in those over 85 years.

Other X-ray signs of CPPD are a "wrapped around" appearance of the patella relative to the femur, and femoral cortical erosions superior to the patella on a lateral view.

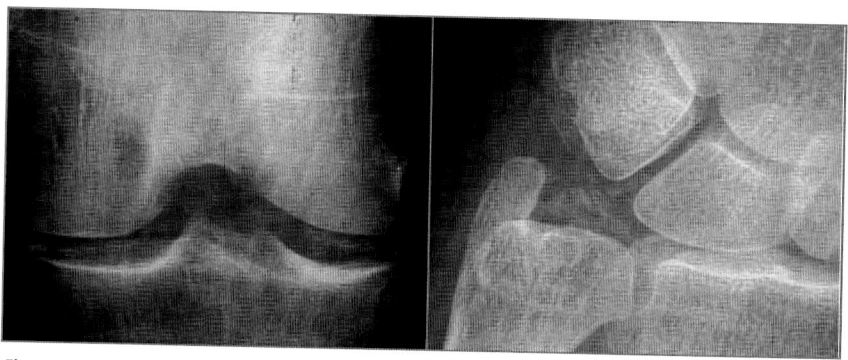

Figure 4. *Chondrocalcinosis. Left panel: This knee X-ray of a patient with pseudogout demonstrates calcium pyrophosphate dihydrate deposition in joint cartilage.*
Manger B, University of Erlangen-Nurnberg, Germany.

Right panel: The triangular ligament of the wrist is another area of predilection for this process. Sometimes the calcification is much more subtle than shown here, and it has to be carefully looked for using a hot lamp.
Filippucci E, Grassi W, University of Ancona, Italy.

What is the best way to diagnose CPPD crystal deposition disease?

Arthrocentesis and synovial analysis with a polarized microscope and first order red compensator is the most important clinical method of diagnosis. A Gram stain and culture of the joint fluid is imperative in pseudogout, as concomitant septic arthritis is possible.

What are the characteristics of the synovial fluid?

The synovial fluid contains rhomboid-shaped, long or short crystals some of which are phagocytized. If viewed under polarized light with a first order red compensator, CPPD crystals demonstrate weakly positive birefringence and shine blue when the long axis of the crystal is parallel to the axis of slow vibration of the compensator. The joint fluid leukocyte count in CPPD crystal deposition disease averages 20,000 per mm^3, as it does in gouty arthritis. The white cell count can be much higher, around 100,000 per mm^3 with over 90% polymorphonuclear leukocytes, a so-called pseudo-septic picture. The joint fluid may be blood-tinged.

Is there effective treatment?

The current mainstay of treatment is a nonsteroidal anti-inflammatory drug. Corticosteroids also have been beneficial, and decreasing the crystal load by arthrocentesis has also shown to be favorable. Treatment of an underlying metabolic disorder does not remove the already formed crystals in the synovial fluid. Colchicine may be effective in prophylaxis.

KEY POINTS

- The acute form of calcium pyrophosphate dihydrate crystal deposition disease is referred to as pseudogout.
- Patients with pseudogout usually present with acute monoarticular arthritis affecting the knees, wrists or metacarpophalangeal joints.
- Synovial fluid contains rhomboid-shaped crystals with weakly positive birefringence.
- The most commonly associated metabolic condition is hyperparathyroidism.
- Treatment consists of an NSAID, and/or arthrocentesis - with injection of a corticosteroid if infection is excluded.

CHAPTER 21

SEPTIC (BACTERIAL) ARTHRITIS

Harold M Adelman

Septic arthritis is a true medical emergency. If appropriate treatment is not started <u>within one week</u> of onset of symptoms, the outlook for joint function and even survival in some cases, is significantly worse. The key to a good outcome is making the right diagnosis promptly and initiating treatment expeditiously! (1).

What is the magnitude of this problem?

The yearly incidence of septic arthritis varies from two to ten per 100,000 in the general population to 30-70 per 100,000 in individuals with rheumatoid arthritis or joint prostheses. A suboptimal functional outcome can be expected in about one third of cases (1).

Which organisms are more commonly responsible for nongonococcal arthritis?

In general 80% of cases of septic arthritis is caused by Gram-positive cocci and 20% by Gram-negative bacilli, though host and environmental factors influence this number significantly. ***Staphylococcus aureus*** is the most frequent cause, and responsible for 60% of cases of nongonococcal septic arthritis, and up to 80% in patients with rheumatoid arthritis or diabetes mellitus. Methicillin-resistant S. aureus occurs in up to 25% of cases, particularly in intravenous drug abusers. Streptococcus species are the etiology in 18% and about 5% are polymicrobial. In England and Wales, 40% of isolates are *S. aureus*, 28% Streptococcal species, and 19% Gram negative bacilli (1).

What are the risk factors for septic arthritis?

Pre-existing joint damage is a major risk factor for septic arthritis, and rheumatoid arthritis is one of the most common causes. In a patient with rheumatoid arthritis, an exacerbation of inflammation in one or a few joints out of phase with the others must be considered as superimposed septic arthritis until proven otherwise by synovianalysis, Gram's stain and culture and sensitivity. Approximately 20% of patients with septic arthritis have rheumatoid arthritis in some series. On the other hand, up to 3% of patients with rheumatoid arthritis will have septic arthritis complicate their disease along the course. In rheumatoid arthritis patients, *S. aureus* is the causative agent in 75% of cases.

Corticosteroids, intraarticular or systemic, are an important cofactor. If a patient with rheumatoid arthritis, or other rheumatic disease, taking a tumor necrosis alpha-blocker develops septic arthritis, or any other infection, this medication must be stopped until the infection is successfully treated. Other arthropathies, including osteoarthritis, also predispose to septic arthritis, and patients with joint arthroplasties and a skin infection are at particular risk. In patients with systemic lupus erythematosus on corticosteroids, septic arthritis can occur with encapsulated organisms, such as *S. pneumoniae or H. influenzae*. Infections with salmonella species are also seen in lupus patients. In fact, the condition most commonly associated with salmonella bacteremia is systemic lupus erythematosus [(2)]. Geographical considerations are exemplified by the higher incidence of tuberculous arthritis in India, and the importance of occupation for brucella arthritis in people who work with animals. Tuberculous arthritis is also increasing pari passu with the AIDS epidemic.

Diseases that suppress the immune system also predispose to septic arthritis. Some examples are diabetes mellitus, chronic liver disease, and patients age 80 years or over. Multiple co-morbidity and advanced age increase the probability of complications and death. A point of interest, joint infections are not common in AIDS. Intravenous drug abuse is another risk factor for septic arthritis and particular joints might be affected. The manubriosternal, acromioclavicular, sternoclavicular, and sacroiliac joints can be involved in intravenous drug abusers, whereas these joints are not usually involved in non-addicts. Brucella infection of the SI joints is an exception.

What is the geographical distribution of organisms causing septic arthritis in intravenous drug abusers?

In the United States, *S. aureus* predominates in the Northeast and in urban centers, *Serratia marcescens* in California, and *Pseudomonas aeruginosa* in some locations in the Midwest. In one study done in Scotland by Gupta et al, 15% of patients with septic arthritis were drug abusers [(3)]. Likewise, in a study in Amsterdam by Kaandorp et al, IV drug abuse was a factor in 9% (14/150) of patients [(4)].

What is the pathophysiology of septic arthritis?

In most cases, hematogenous seeding results in septic arthritis. The synovium is a vascular tissue and does not have a limiting basement membrane. Extension by contiguity results in joint infection in other cases. Tissue damage results from bacterial products as well as host proteolytic enzymes.

How does septic arthritis present clinically?

Septic arthritis typically presents as an acute, hot, very painful joint. In 20% of cases, polyarticular involvement occurs. If the process is occurring in rheumatoid arthritis, it is not unusual for more than one joint to be infected. On physical examination, the joint is obviously inflamed; there is an effusion and marked tenderness. Motion is impeded throughout its range by severe pain.

What other clinical features of septic arthritis are important in diagnosis?

Most patients with septic arthritis are febrile. Fever is seen in about 85% of cases and can be low grade. Patients with a *septic prosthetic joint tend not to have fever*. An infection elsewhere, such as the skin, urinary tract, or lung should heighten one's suspicion of septic arthritis. Joint infection after arthrocentesis or glucocorticoid joint injection is not common, but must be suspected when joint inflammation worsens after such a procedure.

How do the laboratory and radiology help us in diagnosing septic arthritis?

Any patient with acute arthritis of one or two joints of unknown etiology must have an *arthrocentesis and synovianalysis*! If joint fluid cannot be obtained by the usual needle aspiration, the joint should be aspirated under CT, fluoroscopy, or ultrasound guidance. Surgical arthrotomy might be required. The all-important arthrocentesis and synovianalysis reveal an elevated white cell count, typically above 50,000 per mm^3 with >90% polymorphonuclear neutrophils. It is important to note, however, that the synovial fluid white cell count can be lower early in the course of bacterial arthritis, in the first few hours, but the high percentage of neutrophils is still an important clue. Gram's stain of synovial fluid in septic arthritis shows microorganisms in at least 50% of cases and in a higher proportion in S. aureus infection. Thus, a negative Gram's stain does not necessarily rule out septic arthritis. In a patient with acute monoarthritis who has a synovial fluid white count above 50,000 per mm^3, or with more than 90%

polymorphonuclear neutrophils, empiric antibiotics should be instituted until the results of the synovial fluid culture and sensitivity are known! Culture and sensitivity of the joint fluid are positive in over 90% of cases of septic arthritis. A negative joint fluid Gram's stain and culture should be supported by negative joint and blood cultures. In the near future, polymerase chain reaction assay for synovial fluid bacterial DNA will be helpful [5]. Gout or pseudogout can coexist with septic arthritis, so even when crystals are seen, it is important to perform a Gram's stain and culture on synovial fluid. Blood cultures are positive in 50% of cases of septic arthritis, and so should be performed. Peripheral leukocytosis with neutrophilia is common, though not invariable. An elevated erythrosedimentation rate and C-reactive protein are common but nonspecific.

Uncommonly, synovial fluid white cell counts of other arthritides can be as high as 100,000/mm^3, so called pseudoseptic arthritis [6]. Examples are calcium pyrophosphate dihydrate crystal deposition disease, gout, and rheumatoid arthritis. However, septic arthritis complicating these diseases *must* always be presumed until proven otherwise. X-rays of the septic joint appear normal, besides soft tissue swelling, until after the first week. An early film is useful as a baseline or to show contiguous osteomyelitis. Typical joint findings after ten to fourteen days are localized osteopenia, joint space narrowing and erosions. Gas in the joint suggests *E. coli* infection. Magnetic resonance imaging and radionuclide scans are helpful for deep-seated joints such as the hip or sacroiliac joint.

What should we think of in the differential diagnosis of septic arthritis?

Crystal-induced arthritis, e.g. gout and pseudogout, present in a manner very similar to septic arthritis, and importantly, the two conditions can coexist. Demonstration of crystals in synovial fluid neutrophils is diagnostic of the former. A reactive arthritis occasionally presents as acute monoarthritis. Conjunctivitis, uveitis and low back pain help distinguish it, and arthrocentesis and synovianalysis will reveal a lower white cell count and percentage of neutrophils than in septic arthritis. Viral arthritis also is distinguished from septic arthritis by synovianalysis, as well as by viral serology. Lyme arthritis often involves one knee. A history of erythema migrans and living in an area endemic for Lyme disease, with or without a tick bite, assists in the differential diagnosis [7]. Synovianalysis will be helpful, with a white cell count of 10,000 to 25,000/mm^3, mostly neutrophils seen in Lyme arthritis. Synovial fluid cultures are negative in Lyme disease. Rarely, rheumatoid arthritis presents in a similar manner as septic arthritis, with one inflamed joint. Again, Gram's stain and culture of the joint fluid will differentiate between the two. It is important to beware that rheumatoid joints are susceptible to infection! Furthermore, uncommonly one can see a "pseudoseptic" arthritis picture in rheumatoid arthritis, with monarthritis and >100,000 white cells in the joint fluid[(6)].

What factors influence the prognosis of septic arthritis?

Prognosis depends on delay in diagnosis beyond one week, co-morbidity, the initial condition of the joint, and the infecting organism. Staphylococci and gram-negative organisms, for example, are more destructive than streptococci. The mortality rate in adults generally ranges from 10% to 15%. Comorbidity influences this number, especially diabetes mellitus, rheumatoid arthritis, glucocorticoid treatment, chronic liver or renal disease, and active malignancy or AIDS. More than 30% of patients have residual joint damage. This number increases in septic arthritis of the hip.

What are some of the differences between arthritis caused by Neisseria gonorrhoeae and nongonococcal septic arthritis?

Gonococcal (GC) arthritis is the most common septic arthritis in young, healthy, sexually active people in the United States. Women are affected more often, probably because genitourinary infection tends to be asymptomatic more often in women. Because of permissive hormonal changes, the gonococcus is more likely to disseminate during the menses or pregnancy. Factors related to the strain of the organism also contribute to the propensity to disseminate.
GC arthritis is much less frequent in Great Britain. In the United States, GC arthritis accounts for 60% of all septic arthritis; in England and Wales, it accounts for just 0.6%. The reason for this difference is speculative. In the United States, GC arthritis occurs in about 1% of patients with untreated gonorrhea, and in the setting of disseminated infection. However, less GC arthritis has been seen over the past decade in the United States, perhaps because of changing arthritogenicity of gonococcal strains, earlier antibiotic use, and practice of safe sex. In contrast to other bacterial arthritides, GC arthritis is less destructive and usually involves several joints, as a migratory polyarthralgia, initially before settling in one or two joints in the second week[(8)].

The gonococcus, a Gram-negative diplococcus, is a fastidious organism and difficult to grow on culture. Cultures should be plated at bedside on special medium, such as chocolate agar warmed to room temperature, to increase the chances of growing the organism. Cultures of nonsterile areas should be plated on media with antibiotics that inhibit the growth of the normal flora, but not the gonococcus. Examples are Thayer-Martin and New York media. The sample should be transported to the laboratory immediately and incubated in a moist environment of 5% CO2 at 35°C. Even in optimal circumstances, though, the yield from synovial fluid is less than 50%. Gram's stain is positive in less than 25% of patients. Furthermore, the joint fluid white cell count in GC arthritis is lower than in other septic arthritides, usually from 30,000 to 50,000, but reaching 100,000 per mm^3 in some cases. Cultures also should be taken from the cervix, urethra, rectum, pharynx, and a skin lesion if present. The highest yield is from a genitourinary culture, which is positive in about 80% of cases, but it is less specific for GC arthritis. Blood cultures are positive about 10% of the time in GC arthritis. The polymerase chain reaction can identify N. gonorrhoeae and other organisms in culture-negative clinical specimens and might be available in the near future[5].

What are some other features of GC arthritis that are helpful in the differential diagnosis?

Tenosynovitis is frequently seen in GC arthritis, in about two thirds of cases, but not in other bacterial arthritides. Tenosynovitis appears as diffuse swelling of the hand or foot. A particular dermatitis occurs in about one half of patients with disseminated gonococcal infection. It appears as small vesicles, pustules or hemorrhagic macules or bullae. They are few in number and generally appear on the extremities. These lesions are usually not painful, and it is important for the physician to look for them. Their presence argues strongly for the diagnosis of GC arthritis, although similar skin lesions appear in meningococcal arthritis. Tenosynovitis, appearing as disuse swelling of the dorsum of the hand, and the rash tend to occur early in GC arthritis[8].

What is optimal treatment of nongonococcal septic arthritis?

Culture and sensitivity-tailored intravenous antibiotics, and at least daily arthrocenteses to remove injurious bacterial and host products, are the essential elements of treatment. Cidal synovial fluid levels of antibiotics are achieved by intravenous administration. Intra-articular administration of antibiotics is not necessary. For immunocompromised hosts, including those with rheumatoid arthritis, at least four weeks of intravenous antibiotics followed by two weeks of oral therapy is recommended. *Staphylococcal aureus* and Gram-negative species are more injurious to the joint and might require a longer course of treatment. Again, at least daily arthrocenteses is an integral part of treatment of septic arthritis. It is to be emphasized that starting antibiotics must not await the results of synovial fluid culture and sensitivity testing. The choice of initial antibiotic, while awaiting the results of culture and sensitivity testing, depends on the Gram's stain and the clinical aspects of the particular patient. Such aspects include the patient's age, social setting and comorbidity. As a guide to initial antibiotic therapy, if the Gram's stain of synovial fluid is negative, these patient characteristics are useful. For instance, in healthy, young adults, think of gonococci and staphylococci.

If the patient has rheumatoid arthritis and one or two joints flare out of phase with the other joints, think of staphylococci. If the patient is immunocompromised, was recently hospitalized, or is an intravenous drug abuser, organisms to consider include staphylococci, streptococci, and *Pseudomonas*. In an area endemic for Lyme disease, think of *Borrelia*. With a recent dog or cat bite, consider *Pasteurella multocida*. If the patient has symptoms of an infected prosthetic joint, *Staphylococcus epidermidis* and *S. aureus* (possibly methicillin-resistant) are likely. If Gram-positive cocci are identified, treatment should begin with a penicillinase-resistant antibiotic, or vancomycin if there is a penicillin allergy or if methicillin-resistance is suspected. If Gram-negative organisms are present, an aminoglycoside and a third-generation cephalosporin are recommended – if the patient is not allergic to penicillin. If patient is allergic to penicillin, a quinolone is suggested and sensitivity testing is mandatory.

Some specific suggestions follow, (Table 1).

Table 1. Empiric Antibiotic Treatment of Septic Arthritis per Gram-stain and Place of contagion

For community–acquired, hospital-acquired - or nursing home-acquired Gram-positive cocci	vancomycin, (15 mg/kg q12h IV).
Gram's stain shows gram-negative bacilli-	ceftriaxone (2 g IV once daily), ceftazidime (1 to 2 g IV q8h), or cefotaxime (2 g IV q8h). If *Pseudomonas aeruginosa* is suspected, ceftazidime with an aminoglycoside such as gentamicin (7mg/kg IV q6h if renal function is normal). In cephalosporin-allergic patients, ciprofloxacin 400 mg IV every 12 hours.

When joint fluid or blood culture and sensitivity results are available, change antibiotics as indicated.

Synovial fluid white cell counts and cultures should be followed during treatment. If the white cell count is not dropping or the culture remains positive after several days of antibiotic therapy and closed joint drainage, orthopedic consultation and open surgical drainage must be considered. Occasionally, contiguous osteomyelitis is the cause of poor response to treatment. Surgical débridement might be indicated in this case. For the hip or shoulder joints, surgical drainage is probably more effective than closed drainage in removing injurious bacterial and host cell products. In difficult cases, arthroscopic drainage can be advantageous. Joint visualization and thorough irrigation, in slowly improving septic joints, is possible by arthroscopy. When severe pain has abated, gentle range-of-motion exercises are an important adjunct for optimal joint function. Early joint mobilization helps avoid joint contractures. When the patient starts walking, a flare of knee synovitis might occur. If the joint fluid is sterile, treatment with a nonsteroidal anti-inflammatory drug, or if necessary, intraarticular injection of a glucocorticoid, usually suffice.

How is GC arthritis best treated?

The following are our suggestions. As penicillin-resistant and fluoroquinolone-resistant strains of *N. gonorrhoeae* are responsible for many cases of disseminated gonococcal infection (DGI) today, the antibiotic of choice for GC arthritis is ceftriaxone (one g IV or IM q24h). Cefotaxime (one g IV q8h), is an alternative. For cephalosporin- allergic individuals, use spectinomycin (two g IM q12h). Quinolone resistance is on the rise. The CDC recommends at least one week of IV antibiotics, changing to po antibiotics one to two days after clinical improvement is seen. One week of Cefixime (400 mg po bid) is a good choice. If the patient is allergic to cephalosporins, use erythromycin or azithromycin. It is important to treat the patient for concomitant Chlamydial infection with doxycycline (100 mg po every 12 hours for a week), and to treat the patients' sexual partners. Treat asymptomatically infected partners with one dose of ceftriaxone 125 mg IM or cefixime 400 mg orally, in addition to seven days of doxycycline (100 mg po bid) for chlamydial infection. Remember, quinolones and tetracyclines are contraindicated in pregnancy, and erythromycin or azithromycin should be used instead. Concomitant HIV infection also should be ruled out.

Daily joint aspirations are important as long as effusions recur. If follow-up is feasible, the patient can be discharged from the hospital when symptoms have significantly improved; most patients can go home within a week. Response to treatment of GC arthritis is prompt, and the prognosis is excellent.

What are the salient features of infection of the prosthetic joint?

Risk factors for prosthetic joint infection are infection elsewhere in the body, prolonged operative time and delayed wound healing, rheumatoid arthritis, psoriasis, prior joint infection, and corticosteroid therapy. Infection elsewhere in the body must be eradicated before elective arthroplasty is performed. Prosthetic joint infections are considered as early or late. This distinction is of practical importance because the bacteriology and treatment differ. Early prosthetic joint infection, that is, infection *within 12 months* of surgery, is usually caused by intra-operative inoculation of bacteria into the joint or postoperative bacteremia and the patient has persistent joint pain. The frequency of early prosthetic joint infection is less than 2%. The bacteria causing early prosthetic joint infection are *S. aureus* 50%, mixed infections 33%, Gram-negative bacteria 10%, and anaerobes 5%.

On the other hand, late prosthetic joint infection is considered infection occurring *after 12 months* of joint surgery. Pathogenesis is usually bacteremia from infection elsewhere, especially the skin and soft tissue, urinary, and respiratory tracts. The annual rate of late infection is 0.60%. Staphylococcal and streptococcal species account for most of the infections, with *Escherichia coli* and anaerobes making up the remainder. It must be kept in mind that, in early or late prosthetic infection, the process might be insidious. Fever, joint drainage, and swelling are unusual; however, pain and an elevated erythrosedimentation rate and C- reactive protein are the rule. In late infection, distinguishing infection from loosening of the prosthesis can be difficult. However, the possibility of infection always should be kept in mind in the painful prosthetic joint.

Diagnosis of an infected prosthetic joint is made by isolation of the organism by arthrocentesis and synovianalysis or surgical débridement. X-rays are abnormal in half of the cases and show lucency at the bone cement interface, cement fractures and periosteal new bone formation. Scintigraphy is not effective in diagnosing prosthetic joint infections because increased uptake is normally seen for at least six months after arthroplasty, or even with loosening without infection. Treating the infected prosthetic joint is difficult. Most of the time, removal of the prosthesis is necessary, with débridement of all cement and infected tissue followed by a prolonged (six weeks) course of antibiotics. Only about 20% of infected prosthetic hips or knees can be successfully treated without removal of the prosthesis. Immediate or delayed (six weeks) re-implantation of a new prosthesis using antibiotic-impregnated cement is then performed. Re-infection occurs in about 5-10% of cases, but up to 60% if the patient has rheumatoid arthritis, even with meticulous procedure. The necessity of prophylaxis of prosthetic joint infection in procedures causing bacteremia, such as dental work, is unclear; the data do not support one or the other position. Close surveillance after the procedure is wise and orthopedic consultation should be obtained if there is any question of infection.

KEY POINTS

- Septic arthritis is a medical emergency. If treatment is not started within the first week of joint pain, the prognosis for joint function, and even for survival in some cases, is significantly worse.
- The essentials of diagnosing septic arthritis include a high index of suspicion and synovianalysis, with joint fluid Gram's stain, culture and sensitivity, and leukocyte count with differential.
- The most common organisms causing septic arthritis are Staphylococcus aureus, and, in the United States, Neisseria gonorrhoeae in the young, sexually active. In the United Kingdom, arthritis from Neisseria gonorrhoeae is much less common.
- Because of dire consequences if the diagnosis is delayed, septic arthritis must be suspected in any patient presenting with acute arthritis in one joint. Prompt arthrocentesis is imperative and joint fluid examined.
- Even if the Gram's stain is negative, a white cell count of 50,000 or higher, especially with more than 90% polymorphonuclear leukocytes, is suggestive of septic arthritis until proven otherwise by culture.
- Empiric, intravenous antibiotics must be started. Culture and sensitivity results will then direct specific treatment.

- Besides intravenous antibiotics, daily or twice daily joint taps are necessary to remove inflammatory bacterial and host products from the joint.

CHAPTER 22

OTHER INFECTIOUS ARTHRITIDES LYME DISEASE

Harold M. Adelman

Lyme disease is a multisystem, immune-mediated response to infection by the spirochete *Borrelia bergdorferi*, spread by infected Ixodes ticks. Lyme disease is the most common tick-borne disease in the United States. These ticks are also vectors for the agents responsible for human granulocytic ehrlichiosis and for *Babesia microti*, and coinfection occurs. Lyme disease was first described by Steere and Malawista at Yale University[1] after an outbreak in Old Lyme Connecticut in 1977. In Europe, Garin-Bujadour first described the neurologic syndrome of *neuroborreliosis* in the 1920s, and Bannwarth linked it to the characteristic rash, erythema migrans, in 1941. Bannwarth syndrome consists of lymphocytic meningitis, cranial nerve palsy, usually facial, and radiculoneuritis, preceded by a tick bite and erythema migrans.

What are the primary geographical locations and seasons of Lyme disease?

Lyme disease is seen primarily in the North eastern, North central, and Western United States, Europe and Asia. Lyme disease begins in late spring, summer and early fall, so beware of a flu-like illness in these months.

Lyme disease is spread by Ixodes ticks, usually in their nymph stage:

- *scapularis* in the Eastern, North central and Southern United States;
- pacificus in the Western United States;
- ricinus in Europe; and
- persulcatus in Asia.

In the US, adult female ticks feed on white-tailed deer and white-footed mice in autumn and winter, with the blood meal providing the nutrients to make eggs.

What are the clinical manifestations of Lyme disease?

As in another infamous spirochetal disease, syphilis, Lyme disease occurs in three stages: Early localized, early disseminated, and late or chronic Lyme disease [2].

Early Localized Lyme Disease [3]

1. A few days to one month after the tick bite
2. The characteristic rash, erythema migrans (EM), seen in about 50% of patients. EM is found near the axilla, inguinal region, behind the knees, or at the belt line. There sometimes is pruritus or burning. The rash expands for a few days, sometimes with central clearing and a bull's eye appearance. A minority of patients with EM will have several lesions.
3. Fatigue, malaise, headache, stiff neck, muscle and joint pain, lymphadenopathy.

Early Disseminated Lyme Disease

1. Days to 10 months after the tick bite.
2. Carditis, in about 10% of untreated patients
   A) Conduction defects
   B) Arrhythmias
   C) Myo and pericarditis
3. Neurologic disease, in about 10% of untreated patients
   A) Lymphocytic meningitis
   B) Cranial neuropathy, most often facial, can be bilateral
   C) Encephalitis
   D) Radiculoneuropathy
   E) Myelitis
4. Musculoskeletal disease, in about 50% of untreated patients
   A) Migratory polyarthralgias or arthritis
5. Cutaneous disease
   A) Lymphocytoma, a benign lesion on the earlobe or breast
   B) Erythema nodosum
6. Lymphadenopathy

7. Ocular disease
   A) Conjunctivitis
   B) Iritis
   C) Chorioretinitis
   D) Vitreitis

8 Hepatic disease
   A) Elevation of liver enzymes or frank hepatitis

9 Renal disease
   A) Microhematuria
   B) Non-nephrotic proteinuria

Late or Chronic Lyme Disease

1. Months to years after the tick bite

2. Musculoskeletal disease.

   In about 10 % of untreated patients, there is chronic monarthritis, usually affecting a knee. In most individuals, arthritis caused by late Lyme disease resolves with oral antibiotic therapy, intravenous therapy being reserved for arthritis not resolving with oral treatment. In some patients, however, arthritis persists after antibiotic therapy. This is particularly so if the patient has the HLA-D4 haplotype. Persisting arthritis requires treatment with inflammation-suppressing drugs or synovectomy. Physical therapy is helpful for patients with chronic arthritis.

3. Neurologic disease

   A) Prevalence not clear
   B) Subtle changes in mentation
   C) Ataxia
   D) Peripheral neuropathy
   E) Psychiatric disorders
   F) Dementia

4. Cutaneous disease

   Acrodermatitis chronica atrophicans, which are morphea-like skin lesions on the extensor surfaces of the hands, feet, elbows, and knees.

What are the differences in the disease seen in the United States and that seen in Europe?

In the United States, there is a higher frequency of arthritis and multiple erythema migrans lesions. This difference may be due to differences in the organisms, and perhaps to differences in the immunogenetic types of the human hosts [4]. At least three closely related Borrelia species cause Lyme disease. B. burgdorferi *sensu stricto* is the etiologic agent of Lyme disease in the United States, Europe and Asia. B. afzelii and B. garinii also cause Lyme disease in Europe and Asia, but have not been identified in the United States.

How is Lyme disease best diagnosed?

The diagnosis of Lyme disease is made by careful history and physical examination, with strong consideration of the probability of the disease, and *supported by* laboratory serology. Serology is problematic because the methods are not well standardized - in different laboratories or even on the same laboratory [5]. Furthermore, as in all testing in medicine, the pre-test probability of the disease has to be considered to minimize false- positive test results. The pre-test probability of Lyme disease can be approximated by answering these three questions:

- Is Lyme disease known to occur in this area?
- In what season did the tick bite occur?
- Was the tick engorged?

To transmit Lyme disease, a tick has to feed from a human for at least 36 to 48 hours. So, if the tick is not engorged, it did not feed for a time sufficient to transmit Lyme disease. Even in *endemic areas*, the risk of contracting Lyme disease after being bitten by an infected tick is about 4%. In other areas, Lyme disease after a tick bite is not really a practical consideration. Therefore, if serological testing for Lyme disease is done after a tick bite in a nonendemic area, a positive result is highly likely to be a false-positive one.

Therefore, the diagnosis of Lyme disease should be made on the basis of clinical features that strongly propose the diagnosis, and serologic tests should be used only <u>*to confirm*</u> the diagnosis. Moreover, Lyme serology should *not* be used to screen a population. The methods most often used are an enzyme linked immunosorbent assay (ELISA) and Western blot. IgM

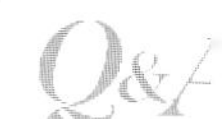

appears two to four weeks after EM, peaks at six to eight weeks, and declines to low levels after four to six months. Thus, serology is often negative in early Lyme disease. IgG appears after six to eight weeks, peaks at four to six months and often remains elevated indefinitely, despite therapy and resolution of symptoms. Unsuccessful treatment early in the course of Lyme disease can cause confusing seronegativity despite progression of the disease. Cross-reactivity and positive ELISA results occur with *Treponema pallidum*, the human granulocytic *Ehrlichia* agent, rheumatoid arthritis and systemic lupus erythematosus, as well as with parvovirus B19 and Epstein-Barr virus. Therefore, Western Blot testing, looking for specific Borrelial antigen bands, should follow positive or unclear ELISA results for *B. burgdorferi*. Furthermore, in nonendemic areas, about five percent of normal people have a false-positive ELISA for *B. burgdorferi*.

Ongoing infection is suggested by sequential Western blot analyses, performed in the same laboratory, demonstrating the appearance of new antigen bands - reactivity with proteins not previously recognized. Worsening or new signs or symptoms should also be present to assume ongoing infection. Polymerase chain reaction for *B. burgdorferi* is being evaluated. Culture of *B. burgdorferi* is usually of low yield, but when positive is diagnostic. EM lesions, heart, cerebrospinal fluid, joint fluid or synovium, and brain can yield positive cultures, depending on the stage of the disease.

How is Lyme Disease Treated?

The best "treatment" is avoidance of tick exposure. If exposure to ticks is unavoidable, use protective clothing and tick repellents, check the entire body for ticks daily, and promptly remove attached ticks before transmission of *B. burgdorferi* can occur. Routine use of antibiotics or serological tests after a tick bite is not recommended. Education of the patient and significant others about the nature and course of Lyme disease is very important. Patients, who are well informed will be less complicated to treat. The choice of specific therapy depends upon the *clinical manifestations*. The Infectious Diseases Society of America (IDSA) has published treatment guidelines [6].

Suggested Antibiotic Regimens for Early, Localized Lyme Disease (in adults)

Doxycycline	100 mg po b.i.d.	Two to three weeks
	<u>Or</u>	
Amoxicillin	500 mg po t.i.d.	Two to three weeks

Early, disseminated and late (chronic) Lyme disease (in adults)[7]

Ceftriaxone	2 g q.d.	Two to four weeks
	<u>Or</u>	
Cefotaxime	3 g b.i.d.	Two to four weeks
	<u>Or</u>	
Penicillin G	20 million units in six divided doses	Two to four weeks

European studies have shown efficacy of oral doxycycline for early neuroborreliosis[8], and mild carditis might be treated effectively with oral antibiotics. A caveat applies: The treatment of neuroborreliosis in Europe might not be the same as that in the United States because of differences in the antigenicity of the infecting organism and the immunogenetic biology of the host.

What is the Jarisch-Herxheimer reaction?

Shortly after starting treatment for Lyme disease, the Jarisch-Herxheimer reaction may occur. This reaction consists of fever, chills, headache, hypotension, and abdominal and pleuritic chest pain, one to two hours after beginning therapy with intravenous antibiotics, particularly penicillin. The reaction is most likely cytokine-mediated, especially by tumor necrosis factor-alpha and interleukins-6 and -8. The Jarisch-Herxheimer reaction can be mitigated by antipyretics or with the careful use of glucocorticoids.

What is the prognosis of Lyme Disease?

The earlier it is treated, the better the prognosis. Even in late disease, prognosis is good with appropriate antibiotic treatment.

Who Should Get Vaccinated Against B. Burgdorferi?

A recombinant outer surface protein A (OspA) vaccine against Lyme disease is now in use in the US. The vaccine is derived from a lipidated outer surface protein of *Borrelia burgdorferi*. Its mechanism is unique because it works *inside* the tick vector, rendering the organism noninfective [9, 10]. The United States Advisory Committee on Immunization Practices (ACIP) has recommended that "vaccination should be considered for patients 15 to 70 years of age who live, work, and recreate in high- or moderate-risk areas, and are exposed to ticks either frequently or for long periods of time." It should be noted that the heterogeneity of many Borrelial proteins, for example, OspC in Europe, will require different vaccines for different parts of Europe.

KEY POINTS

- Lyme disease is a multisystem disease caused by the spirochete Borrelia burgdorferi and transmitted by the Ixodes tick.
- The disease occurs on multiple continents.
- There are three stages of Lyme disease: Early localized, early disseminated and late or chronic Lyme disease.
- Diagnosis is problematic at this time because of nonstandardized serologic tests.
- The history and physical examination, with strong consideration of the pre-serologic probability of the disease, are the linchpins of diagnosis. Serology is confirmative.
- Treatment consists of antibiotics, and varies according to the stage of the disease.
- With appropriate antibiotic treatment, the prognosis of Lyme disease is usually good.

TUBERCULOUS ARTHRITIS

Tuberculosis is on the rise again, probably because of the AIDS epidemic as well as travel to and from developing countries. Furthermore, tumor necrosis factor alpha blocker therapy can reactivate latent tuberculosis. Musculoskeletal manifestations of Mycobacterium tuberculosis infection include tuberculous arthritis as well as tuberculous spondylitis (Pott's disease), osteomyelitis, tenosynovitis, and a reactive arthritis known as Poncet's disease, from M. tuberculosis or M. avium complex infection elsewhere in the body[(1)]. Intra-bladder therapy with Bacillus Calmette-Guérin (BCG) vaccine of bladder cancer can cause a reactive arthritis too. One of the multiple causes of erythema nodosum is infection with M. tuberculosis.

Tuberculous arthritis is an insidious condition of one joint, usually a knee or hip. There is painful swelling, but other signs of inflammation are minor, leading to delay in diagnosis. Furthermore, the chest X-ray is negative in more than half of the cases. The synovial fluid white cell count is in the range of 500-50,000 cells/mm^3, usually predominantly neutrophils. Acid-fast stain of synovial fluid is usually negative, and culture of synovial fluid can be negative in about 30 % of cases. The polymerase chain reaction assay of synovial fluid can yield rapid results. Non-specific rheumatoid factor positivity can occur in tuberculous arthritis. PPD is usually positive, unless the patient is anergic from glucocorticoid therapy or AIDS. Tuberculous arthritis can be a presenting manifestation of AIDS. Joint X-rays reveal nonspecific soft tissue swelling, periarticular osteopenia, joint erosions, and joint space narrowing from cartilage destruction. There is also periostitis.

Fungal arthritis is in the differential diagnosis. Diagnosis of tuberculous arthritis is best made by culture and histology of synovial tissue, which shows caseating or noncaseating granulomata. These studies are positive in about 95% of cases. Regarding therapy, one regimen is isoniazid and rifampin for nine months[(2)]. Ethambutol should be given in addition for the first two months of treatment. The possibility of multi-drug resistance should be kept in mind, and consultation with an infectious disease specialist is warranted. Concomitant HIV disease must be considered. Surgical consultation is indicated for possible joint debridement or synovectomy.

VIRAL ARTHROPATHIES

Can viruses cause arthritis?

Various viruses can cause arthralgias or arthritis lasting weeks [1]. Parvovirus B19 [2], the HIV [3], hepatitis B and C [4, 5], rubella, mumps, Chikungunya – Swahili for, "That which bends up," and O'nyong-nyong – Ugandan Acholi dialect for "Joint breaker," among other viruses, are arthritogenic.

Why is it important to know about parvovirus B19 infection?

This common infection can closely mimic rheumatoid arthritis and systemic lupus erythematosus [6]. In adults, infection with Parvovirus B19 differs from the classic fifth disease, or erythema infectiosum, in children. In adults, the characteristic bright red "slapped-cheek" rash is not usually seen. On the other hand, joint involvement occurs more frequently with advancing age. The pattern of joint involvement in Parvovirus B19 infection is a sudden onset of symmetric polyarthritis (five or more joints), involving the proximal interphalageal and metatarsophalangeal joints, the wrists, knees and ankles. There is morning stiffness. The arthritis usually abates over several weeks; however, some patients have joint involvement for months or years. The arthritis can be intermittent and joint destruction does not occur [7, 8, 9]. Treatment of Parvovirus B19 arthritis is with NSAIDs and physical/occupation therapy.

Parvovirus B19 infection is the most common cause of pure red cell aplasia in AIDS patients [10]. Bone marrow examination shows the tell-tale giant pronormoblast. Further, in patients with compensated hemolytic anemia, such as those with sickle cell disease, infection with parvovirus B19 can cause pure red cell aplasia or pancytopenia. For severe cases of bone marrow disfunction, treatment with intravenous immunoglobulin can be helpful.

Therefore, parvovirus B19 infection can closely imitate rheumatoid arthritis [11], including a positive rheumatoid factor early in the course, and systemic lupus erythematosus, with the hematologic involvement and the serologies – including a positive ANA and even a positive double-stranded DNA [6, 12]. However, there are no giant pronormoblasts in the marrow of patients with systemic lupus erythematosus.

What about HIV?

HIV affects the joints in several ways[3]. One condition, a very painful polyarthritis called The Painful Articular Syndrome, can require narcotic analgesics. Hospitalization might be warranted. There is no synovitis, and the arthralgias last about 24 hours. The Painful Articular Syndrome can be the initial expression of infection with HIV. Another joint problem unique to HIV infection is HIV-Associated Arthritis. This is an asymmetrical oligo- or polyarthritis lasting less than six weeks. Joint fluid white cell count is usually non-inflammatory, between 500 and 2000/ul, and Gram's stain and culture are negative. Treatment includes NSAIDs, hydroxychloroquine or sulfasalazine. HIV infection can exacerbate psoriatic arthritis.

CHAPTER 23

RS3PE (REMITTING SERONEGATIVE SYMMETRIC SYNOVITIS WITH PITTING EDEMA)

Harold M Adelman

Is this a cousin of R2D2 of Star Wars' fame?

No, RS3PE, or **R**emitting, **S**eronegative, **S**ymmetric **S**ynovitis with **P**itting **E**dema (note that the S's are in alphabetical order) is an inflammatory disorder affecting people over the age of 50. As the name implies, the condition is self-limited, rheumatoid factor and antinuclear antibody negative, and characterized by a dramatic, mitten-like swelling of the hands[(1)]. Etiopathogenesis is unclear.

How does this syndrome present?

There is acute pitting edema of the dorsa of the hands; some patients can even state the date and time of onset. There is also synovitis of the wrists and flexor tendons of the fingers. The feet and knees can be involved as well.

How is RS3PE treated?

This syndrome responds well to low dose prednisone, 10 mg a day. An alternative tact, that does not act as promptly, is hydroxychloroquine and a nonsteroidal anti-inflammatory drug.

What is the prognosis of RS3PE?

Complete and lasting remission usually occurs within one year, although slight flexion contractures of the fingers and wrists are common. A minority of patients have a few relapses, and a few have been reported to eventuate as rheumatoid arthritis or a spondyloarthropathy[(2)].

Can RS3PE be associated with malignancy?

Yes, in some cases RS3PE is a paraneoplastic syndrome. This possibility should be suspected if the disease does not respond to glucocorticoid treatment [3] or if there is fever or weight loss. Lymphoma, myelodysplastic syndrome, and adenocarcinomas are associated with RS3PE [4].

KEY POINTS

- RS3PE stands for remitting seronegative symmetrical synovitis with pitting edema.
- RS3PE is characterized by diffuse, pitting edema of the dorsa of the hands, so - called mitten hands - bilaterally, and less often of the feet.
- This condition is sometimes associated with an internal malignancy.
- Features suggestive of such are fever and weight loss.
- RS3PE is very responsive to low dose predinsone, 10 mg qam. Failure to respond to a glucocorticoid is also suggestive of related malignancy.
- The prognosis of this condition is excellent. As the name tells us, this disease remits. Occasionally, there is some residual stiffness of the hand joints.

CHAPTER 24

FIBRODYSPLASIA (MYOSITIS) OSSIFICANS PROGRESSIVA

Harold M Adelman

What is fibrodysplasia ossificans progressiva?

Fibrodysplasia ossificans progressiva, or Munchmeyer's disease, is a chronic, progressive, diffuse ossification of the musculature [1]. It is an autosomal dominant disease, beginning in childhood as warm, tender swelling in the muscles of the back of the neck and shoulders. Ossification ensues, and the musculature of the abdomen, chest and extremities become involved. If the swelling is close to a joint, the condition simulates acute arthritis [2].

What are the associated congenital defects that assist in diagnosis?

Interesting associated congenital defects are a short great toe and thumb, exostoses, a broad femoral neck, absence of the two upper incisors, hypogenitalism, absence of the ear-lobes, and deafness [3]. Sometimes, a parent will have just one of these associated anomalies, such as a short great toe.

What course does this disease take?

There can be calcification across joints resulting in ankylosis. Eventually, bone replaces muscle, tendons, fascia, and ligaments, and motion in that particular region is lost.

Is there any treatment for this disease?

A diphosphonate, ethane-1-hydroxy-1, 1-diphosphonate (EHDP) can halt the ossification of newer lesions by preventing the crystal growth of hydroxyapatite and the deposition of calcium phosphate [4]. Its effect on established lesions is poor.

KEY POINTS

- Fibrodysplasia Ossificans Progressiva is a widespread condition of connective tissue that is inherited in an autosomal dominant pattern.
- The condition usual begins in childhood.
- There is tender swelling in several sites that becomes hardened as the lesions ossify. These lesions can come and go.
- Associated anomalies include a short great toe or thumb, absence of the two upper incisors, absence of the ear-lobes, or deafness.
- Treatment with ethane-1-hydroxy-1, 1-diphosphonate (EHDP) can stop progression of early lesions in some patients.
- The prognosis of this disease is poor, however, because of the occurrence of restrictive lung disease and respiratory failure.

CHAPTER 25

REFLEX SYMPATHETIC DYSTROPHY (COMPLEX REGIONAL PAIN SYNDROME TYPE I)

Bryan A Bognar

What causes reflex (RSD)?

An exaggerated response to injury, allowing changes in pain signaling and regulation, are thought to lead to this syndrome. The end result is the generation of pain signals or an exaggerated response to stimuli. The time from the initial inciting event to the initial development of RSD symptoms may be as short as a few days or as long as six months. In most cases, but not all, an inciting event can be identified. Trauma, which can be trivial, crush injuries, contusions, surgery, chemical and electrical burns, and malignancies are antecedents. Myocardial infarction and stroke are also well known precursors.

Are there other names for RSD?

RSD has a large number of synonyms, including among others causalgia, shoulder-hand syndrome, Sudeck's atrophy, sympathalgia, algodystrophy, and hyperpathic pain. A new term, complex regional pain syndrome (Type 1) has become increasingly used.

How is RSD diagnosed?

RSD is a clinical and radiographic diagnosis. There is no universally accepted definition, but several criteria have been offered [4]. The following criteria are helpful in diagnosing RSD:

- **Definite RSD:** pain associated with allodynia (pain from light touch) or hyperpathia (pain persisting or increasing after light touch), tenderness, vasomotor changes, dystrophic skin changes, and swelling
- **Probable RSD:** pain associated with allodynia or hyperpathia, vasomotor changes, and swelling
- **Possible RSD:** vasomotor changes and swelling alone.

What is the Steinbroker staging system for RSD?

Steinbrocker and Argyros described three stages in RSD[5] (Table one). Some authors have included a fourth stage.

Table 1. Reflex Sympathetic Dystrophy (Complex Regional Pain Syndrome Type I)

Stage one	The acute stage, characterized by pain, swelling, and vasomotor changes: there is a dusky purple color with dependent rubor of the involved extremity. Temperature can be increased or decreased.
Stage two	The dystrophic stage, characterized by continued pain and the development of brawny edema and atrophy of the skin.
Stage three	The atrophic stage, characterized by atrophy of the subcutaneus tissue, stiffening of the skin and soft tissues, with contractures. The skin will frequently have a shiny, smooth, tight appearance.
Some authors offer a fourth stage	The psychological stage recognizes the frequency with which these patients develop severe depression and adjustment problems.

However, other authorities have questioned the clinical utility of the staging system. Patients often migrate between stages one and two over a long period of time. In addition, there is considerable variability in the length of time a patient might spend in any given stage. Finally, the dividing lines between stages are not always clear and individual patients may not easily fit into one distinct stage.

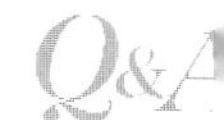

What about radiology and the clinical laboratory in RSD?

X-rays show a patchy, mottled osteopenia (Sudeck's atrophy) of the affected part in most patients with RSD. Nuclide scintigraphy is suggestive, with increased uptake in the involved area [6]. The laboratory is noncontributory. The erythrosedimentation rate, C-reactive protein, and other acute phase reactants are normal, unless there is another reason for them to be elevated.

What are the typical clinical features of RSD?

The usual clinical manifestations of RSD include painful swelling, usually in a distal extremity, accompanied by trophic skin changes and signs or symptoms of vasomotor and sudomotor instability. Vasodilation or vasoconstriction, with consequent increased or decreased temperature and a dusky purple color and dependent rubor of the extremity characterize the vasomotor instability. Hyperhidrosis - increased sweating and hypertrichosis, increased hair, typify the sudomotor abnormalities. A localized increase in sweating is very suggestive of RSD. The pain of RSD is characteristically burning in nature, constant, and intense. This type of pain is referred to as "causalgia". If left untreated, RSD can progress to dystrophic, shiny skin and brittle nails with resultant atrophy and contractures, which may eventuate to a Dupuytren's-like hand.

Can you prevent RSD from developing?

There is no conclusive evidence that RSD can be prevented, especially following fracture or traumatic nerve injury, but early mobilization or physical therapy of the affected limb seems to be beneficial.

Which parts of the body are most frequently affected by RSD?

Involvement of the entire hand, "mitten hand", or foot is the most common presentation, although a radial form involving one or two fingers or toes has been described. Much less common, short segments of bone, the hip, or the knee may be involved. The frequency with which the ipsilateral shoulder is involved when a hand is affected by RSD fostered the term "shoulder-hand syndrome."

Once suspected, how do you treat early RSD?

Most often, the initial treatment of early RSD consists of analgesic agents, such as NSAIDs, in addition to physical modalities including range of motion exercises as tolerated, strengthening exercises, heat/ice, and contrast baths. This conservative approach is generally recommended for the first four weeks. If the patient fails to respond, a more aggressive approach is warranted and may include sympathetic blockade via injection. Surgical sympathectomy is then used in those who have responded to a trial of injection blockade. Many rheumatologists favor a trial of oral corticosteroids [(1)]. It is unclear how corticosteroids work in RSD . Peripherally distributed N-methyl-D-aspartate (NMDA) receptors are important in processing nociceptive information. Ketamine gel, which blocks NMDA receptors, has been studied and might be effective for early, acute RSD [(7)].

Are there any treatments for late stage or atrophic RSD?

Yes, but they are of limited success late in the course of RSD. Therefore, treatment goals shift toward maximizing pain relief and minimizing disability. Spinal cord stimulation is an option for chronic, recalcitrant RSD [(8)]. Treatment is no different than for other chronic, neuropathic pain syndromes; however, in some cases, amputation is required for relief of pain.

KEY POINTS

- RSD is a pain syndrome, most commonly resulting from trauma to an extremity.
- RSD is diagnosed clinically and radiographically.
- Early clinical features include diffuse swelling and burning pain, accompanied by signs or symptoms of vasomotor and sudomotor instability.
- RSD is treated with early physical therapy, including range of motion exercises as tolerated.
- Systemic corticosteroids and sympathetic nerve blocks also have been used successfully.

SECTION FOUR

MISCELLANEOUS RHEUMATIC CONDITIONS

CHAPTER 26

CARPAL TUNNEL SYNDROME

Harold M Adelman

Carpal tunnel syndrome is the most frequent reason for paresthesias of the hand [1]. There are various predisposing conditions that narrow the carpal tunnel in the wrist, with consequent impingement of the median nerve (Figure 1).

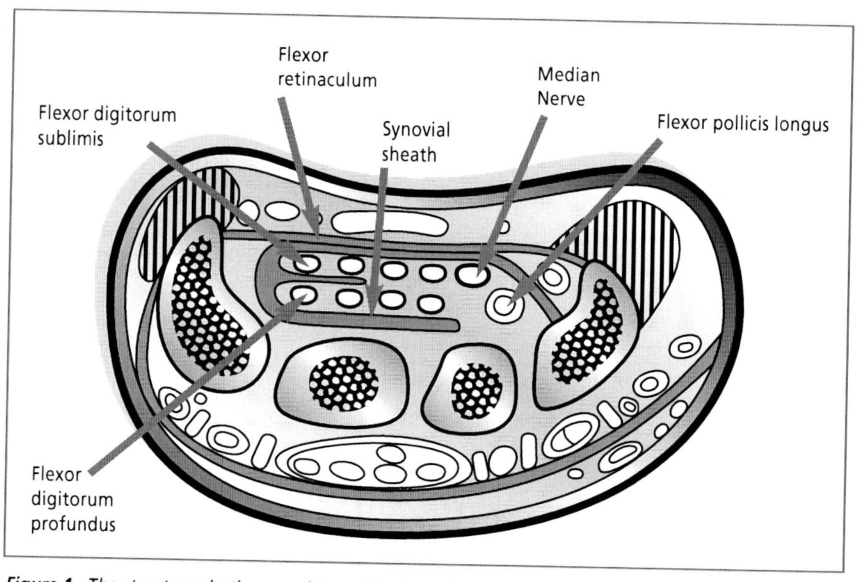

Figure 1. *The structures in the carpal tunnel in the wrist. Note that the median nerve is impinged on when there is swelling of the components of the carpal tunnel.*

Some conditions that cause carpal tunnel syndrome are rheumatoid arthritis, gout, deposition of amyloid L protein (primary amyloidosis and amyloidosis related to multiple myeloma), diabetes mellitus – as part of diabetic neuropathy - pregnancy, jackhammer workers, and excessive typing. Myxedema and acromegaly have been associated with carpal tunnel syndrome [2]. Many cases are idiopathic. Signs and symptoms of carpal tunnel syndrome are tingling or painful paresthesias in the median nerve distribution, that is, the first three fingers and the radial half of the fourth finger. Maneuvers that elicit these symptoms of carpal tunnel syndrome are tapping gently over the volar wrist, Tinel sign, and maintaining the wrists in palmar flexion for one minute, Phalen sign. Typically, the paresthesias in carpal tunnel syndrome are worse at night and when the hands are draped over the steering wheel of a car – a sort of "auto-auto" Phalen sign. There is weakness of the thenar muscles, with impaired flexion, opposition and abduction of the innervated fingers. The paresthesias can extend above the wrist to the elbow, and bilateral involvement is not unusual. Diagnosis is differentiated from similar symptoms caused by radiculopathy from cervical spondylosis with electrodiagnotic studies showing prolonged distal latency.

Treatment of carpal tunnel syndrome entails a wrist splint in the neutral position, and injection of a glucocorticoid into the carpal tunnel using a 25-gauge needle and the palmar approach. Care should be exercised to avoid the median nerve. If these maneuvers fail, surgery is indicated to release the transverse carpal ligament (flexor retinaculum) (Figure 1). When there is atrophy of the thenar eminence in the carpal tunnel syndrome, surgical release of the transverse carpal ligament is indicated.

CHAPTER 27

POPLITEAL (BAKER'S) CYST

Edward P Cutolo

What is a popliteal cyst?

A popliteal cyst, also known as a Baker's cyst, is a synovial fluid collection that accumulates behind the knee joint in the semimembranosus-gastrocnemius bursa. About 40% of the population have a one-way valve-like mechanism between the knee and this bursa [(1)]. An asymptomatic cystic (Figure 1) swelling behind the knee may be the initial manifestation, which can eventually enlarge and cause pain as the synovium becomes inflamed [(1)].

What conditions are associated with a Baker's cyst?

Osteoarthritis, rheumatoid arthritis or any other internal derangement of the knee associated with increased intraarticular pressure is associated with the formation of a Baker's cyst [(1)].

What is the pathophysiology of the formation of the Baker's cyst?

Increased intraarticular pressure from effusion predisposes to Baker's cyst.

What is the pseudothrombophlebitis syndrome?

Physicians must be aware that a Baker's cyst can dissect down the calf or rupture. Pain, swelling, and erythema of the calf, and occasionally edema of the ankle, sometimes even with fever and leukocytosis, caused by a Baker's cyst dissecting down the calf mimic a deep vein thrombophlebitis (figure 1), and characterize the pseudothrombophlebitis syndrome [(2)].

When a Baker's cyst ruptures, blood can settle around a malleolus causing the so-called "crescent sign": a crescent of ecchymosis about a malleolus.

How is the diagnosis of pseudothrombophlebitis established?

Noninvasive vascular studies, such as duplex ultrasound as performed in the evaluation of deep venous thrombosis, is useful in establishing the

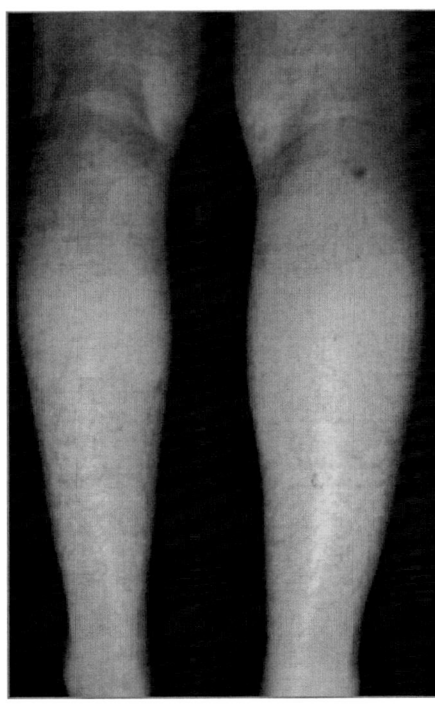

Figure 1. Ruptured popliteal cyst. The fluid has leaked down the soft tissue of the right leg mimicking a deep vein thrombophlebitis. Note that the right calf is larger than the left.

Grassi W. University of Ancona, Italy.

diagnosis of a dissecting Baker's cyst (Figure 2). Venography or duplex ultrasound can be used to exclude concomitant thrombophlebitis. Patients with a Baker's cyst are at risk of developing a true deep venous thrombosis because of venous stasis caused by the cyst [1].

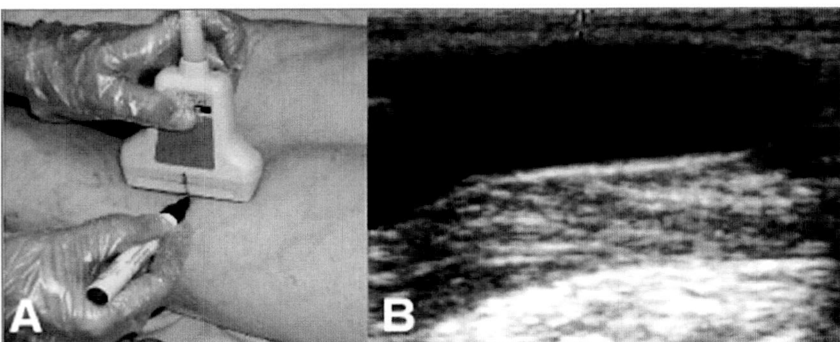

Figure 2. Ultrasonography of the knee. A: Posterior longitudinal scan. B: Ultrasound examination detects an anechoic fluid collection indicating the presence of a popliteal cyst.

Koski J. Mikkeli Central Hospital, Finland.

How is a Baker's cyst treated?

If the Baker's cyst is secondary to an inflammatory arthritis, a corticosteroid injection into the knee joint may suffice. If the cyst is from internal derangement of the knee, surgical repair of the knee is often necessary to prevent recurrence [1].

KEY POINTS

- A Baker's cyst represents swelling from fluid collection in the semimembranosus-gastrocnemius bursa.
- A Baker's cyst results from increased pressure in the knee joint from any cause, and/or an effusion in the semimembranosus-gastrocnemius bursa per se.
- Squatting, with attendant increased intraarticular pressure, is a common antecedent.
- The patient feels fullness behind the knee.
- A Baker's cyst can mimic or even cause deep vein thrombophlebitis.
- Treatment involves aspiration of and injection of a glucocorticoid into the knee joint.

CHAPTER 28

OTHER BURSITIDES AND TENDINITIDES

Bryan B Bognar

How does bursitis/tendonitis usually develop?

Bursitis and tendonitis (tenosynovitis) refer to the inflammation of either a bursal sac or tendinous sheath, respectively. Both commonly result from either trauma or repetitive activities (micro-trauma). On occasion, bursitis/tendonitis can result from another disorder, such as rheumatoid arthritis or gout [1].

What are the most common forms of bursitis?

- Trochanteric bursitis of the hip
- Subacromial or subdeltoid bursitis of the shoulder
- Olecranon bursitis of the elbow
- Prepatellar bursitis ("housemaid's knee" or "wrestler's knee")
- Achilles bursitis ("pump bumps")
- Calcaneal bursitis ("policeman's heel")
- Bunion of the great toe
- Ischial bursitis ("weaver's bottom")
- Anserine bursitis of the knee
- Iliopectineal (or iliopsoas) bursitis
- Obturator internus bursitis.

Can a bursa get infected?

Yes it can. The signs of a septic bursitis are pain and increased warmth of the bursa. There is an increased white blood cell count in the bursal fluid as well as a diagnostic Gram's stain and culture and sensitivity. Infectious bursitis has to be treated with the appropriate antibiotic. The most commonly infected bursae are the olecranon and pre-patellar bursae [2].

What is the treatment of bursitis?

Therapy of bursitis typically consists of a combination of approaches. First, it is important that the patient limit further irritation or trauma. This may require a change of work activities or the simple addition of appropriate padding. A mainstay of therapy is a nonsteroidal anti-inflammatory drug (NSAID); many find local heat and physical therapy with ultrasound to be beneficial. Ice might be effective in the very acute stage. At the same time, a local injection of a corticosteroid is beneficial for non-septic bursitis, although, complications such as skin atrophy should be considered. It is to be emphasized that a shorter acting corticosteroid is less likely to cause skin atrophy. For septic bursitis, the appropriate antibiotic is, of course, the proper treatment.

What are the most common forms of tendinitis?

The most common forms of tendinitis include:

- Lateral epicondylitis ("tennis elbow")
- Medial epicondylitis ("golfer's elbow")
- Bicipital tendonitis
- Rotator cuff tendinitis (especially supraspinatus tendonitis) (Figure 1)
- Tenosynovitis of the wrist
- Patellar tendinitis ("jumper's knee")

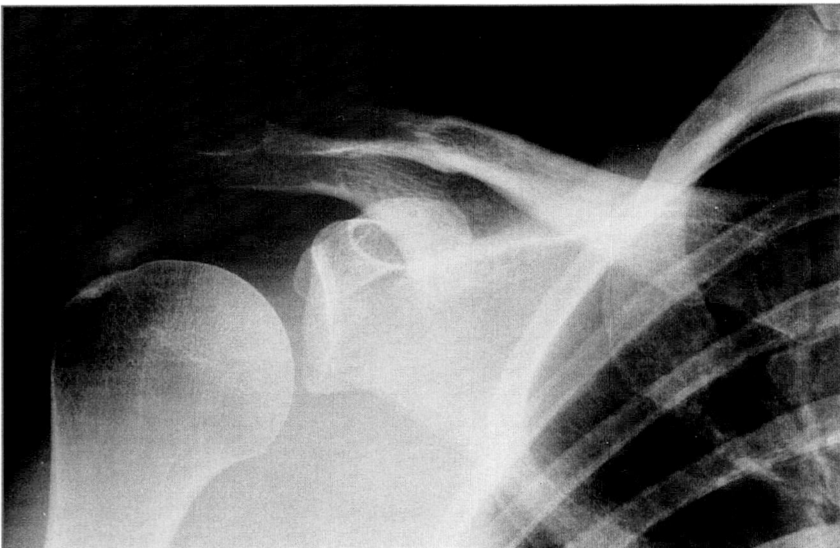

Figure 1. *An X-ray of this patient's right shoulder shows calcification of the supraspinatus tendon.*

What is the treatment for tendinitis?

As with bursitis, many cases of tendonitis result from repetitive activities often related to work or sports. Therapy consists of appropriate reductions in aggravating activities, in addition to an NSAID. Locally applied ice, heat, and physical therapy including ultrasound have also been utilized. Local injections of a short acting corticosteroid are typically reserved for a hyperacute case or those not responding to the above modalities.

How are tendinitis and bursitis diagnosed?

The history and physical examination typically allow diagnosis. Pain in the affected bursa or tendon with movement or palpation is almost universal. Radiologic studies are supportive but non-specific; calcification in the area of a bursa or tendon is indicative.

What is the prognosis of tendinitis and bursitis?

The prognosis of most cases of bursitis or tendonitis is excellent with appropriate treatment. Unfortunately, recurrence is common and a few patients go on to develop more chronic inflammation and calcification requiring surgery.

KEY POINTS

- Both bursitis and tendinitis typically result from either discrete trauma or repetitive activities such as sports (micro-trauma).
- Both bursitis and tendinitis are clinical diagnoses, although X-rays often, but not invariably, indicate soft tissue calcification corresponding to the bursa or tendon.
- Therapy consists of rest, heat/ice, NSAIDs, and for more severe cases, locally injected, short - acting corticosteroids unless the bursa is infected. Surgical bursectomy might be necessary for particularly recalcitrant cases.
- Range of motion exercises and physical therapy as appropriate are beneficial, and can prevent a frozen shoulder (adhesive capsulitis).
- The prognosis is generally excellent, although recurrences occur.

CHAPTER 29

SELECTED DERMATO – ARTHRITIDES SYNDROMES

ERYTHEMA NODOSUM

Harold M Adelman

What is erythema nodosum?

Erythema nodosum (EN) is a skin condition caused by inflammation of the septa of fat lobules. It is thus a septal panniculitis, and not a vasculitis. Most cases of EN are idiopathic, but it can represent an early sign of a variety of infections [1]. Streptococcus, Mycobacterium tuberculosis, deep fungal infections, and Yersinia are infectious agents associated with EN. Sarcoidosis, inflammatory bowel disease, Behçet's syndrome, and medications such as oral contraceptives and sulfa drugs are also related to EN. When associate with sarcoidosis and hilar lymphadenopathy, so-called Lofgren's syndrome, EN indicates an excellent prognosis of the sarcoidosis. Recurring lesions usually indicate an underlying disease, and an investigation is warranted. A recent article from Spain discusses some of these features [2].

What about the pathogenesis of EN?

Pathogenesis probably involves a delayed hypersensitivity reaction to antigens associated with the various infectious agents discussed above, drugs or unknown etiologies.

What are the clinical manifestations of EN?

EN most often affects women from 15 to 40 years of age. EN presents as painful red or violaceous subcutaneous nodules, usually involving the pretibial regions. Sometimes these nodules are easier palpated than seen. As they age, the nodules appear ecchymotic and resolve without scarring (Figure one). Systemic symptoms such as polyarthralgias, fever, and general malaise occur. Acute phase reactants are usually elevated.

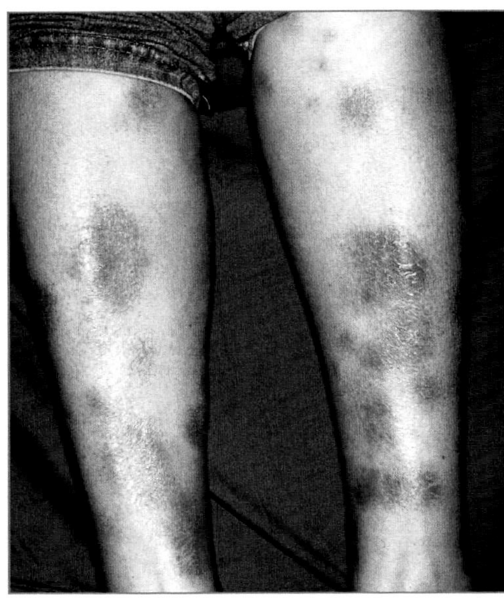

Figure 1. This patient with sarcoidosis had bilateral hilar lymphadenopathy, erythema nodosum, and arthritis, a combination known as Lofgren's syndrome.

How is EN treated?

Nonsteroidal antiinflammatory drugs can be effective. EN is very responsive to glucocorticoids, if they are not contraindicated by an associated condition. Treating the underlying condition can be effective. EN usually resolves in a few weeks even without treatment.

How is EN treated?

Nonsteroidal antiinflammatory drugs can be effective. EN is very responsive to glucocorticoids, if they are not contraindicated by an associated condition. Treating the underlying condition can be effective. EN usually resolves in a few weeks even without treatment.

KEY POINTS

- Erythema nodosum (EN) is a subcutaneous reaction pattern to an antigen.
- Most cases of EN are idiopathic, but infections, medications and other diseases can be associated with EN.

- Painful, red to violet nodules, most often in a pretibial distribution, characterize EN. These nodules evolve though a bruise-like coloration before fading in a few weeks.
- Arthralgias, fever and malaise are extracutaneous manifestations of EN.
- Nonsteroidal antiinflammatory drugs, glucocorticoids, and treatment of an underlying disease are effective therapies.

SWEET'S SYNDROME (ACUTE FEBRILE NEUTROPHILIC DERMATOSIS)

What is Sweet's syndrome?

Sweet's syndrome, or acute febrile neutrophilic dermatosis, is a dermato-arthritis syndrome characterized by painful, erythematous plaques with a predilection for the head, neck, and upper extremities. It is not a vasculitis. Arthritis occurs in about a quarter of patients and is characterized by acute, self-limited polyarthritis[(1)]. Sweet's syndrome can be confused with SLE or erythema nodosum. Treatment is with NSAIDs, and glucocorticoids in moderate doses can be very effective. The majority of cases of Sweet's syndrome are idiopathic, but malignancies (15%), particularly acute myelogenous leukemia, myelodysplastic syndrome, and drug-associated cases, e.g., granulocyte colony-stimulating factor or sulfa drugs, have been reported[(2)]. Thus, careful systemic evaluation with particular attention to blood parameters is important in Sweet's syndrome.

KEY POINTS

- Sweets syndrome, also known as acute febrile neutrophilic dermatosis, is characterized clinically by painful, erythematous plaques with a predilection for the head, neck, and upper extremities.
- Arthritis occurs in about a quarter of patients and is characterized by an acute, self-limited polyarthritis.

- Most cases are idiopathic, but malignancies are associated in about 15% of cases of Sweet's syndrome, most commonly acute myelogenous leukemia.
- Treatment is with NSAIDs, and glucocorticoids in moderate doses can be very effective for resistant cases.

MULTICENTRIC RETICULOHISTIOCYTOSIS

What is this rare form of destructive arthritis?

Multicentric reticulohistiocytosis is a multisystem disease of unknown etiology affecting primarily the joints and skin. Pathogenesis involves infiltration of tissue by glycolipid-laden histiocytes and multinucleated giant cells[(1)]. Multicentric reticulohistiocytosis might be a form of lipid storage disease.

How does this arthropathy present?

In about 60% of cases, multicentric reticulohistiocytosis presents as a symmetrical polyarthritis, involving five or more joints, including the small joints of the hands. The distal interphalangeal joints are often involved. Spinal subluxations can occur. Skin nodules and papules usually follow joint involvement, and take a characteristic bead-like pattern around the nail folds – the so-called "coral bead" appearance. The nodules are yellowish, purple or brown. Nodules on the elbows and face occur, as can oral, nasal, and pharyngeal ulcers. In 40% of cases, skin involvement occurs with the disease, or preceding the arthritis.

Which two, more common, arthritides characteristically involve the distal interphalangeal joints?

Osteoarthritis and psoriatic arthritis have a propensity to involve the distal interphalangeal joints of the hands. Erosive, or inflammatory, osteoarthritis can cause destructive changes of the DIP joints. Adult onset Still's disease can also affect the distal interphalageal joints of the hands.

How can you tell the difference between joint swelling from synovitis of the distal interphalangeal joints (multicentric reticulohistiocytosis or psoriatic arthritis) and joint swelling from osteophyte formation (osteoarthritis)?

Joint swelling from synovitis feels boggy, doughy or spongy on palpation, whereas joint swelling from osteophyte formation feels hard.

What other organ involvement can occur in this multisystem disease?

Pleuritis and pleural effusion, pericarditis, and cardiac conduction defects can be seen with multicentric reticulohistiocytosis, as well as gastrointestinal involvement.

What are the laboratory and radiographic findings?

Laboratory findings are nonspecific. Rheumatoid factor and antinuclear antibodies are not present. The erythrosedimentation rate is elevated in about a third of patients. Synovial fluid white cell counts range widely, from <1,000 to about 30,000 cells per mm^3, mostly mononuclear cells. A Wright-stained smear or wet preparation of synovial fluid might reveal giant cells of large macrophages. X-ray studies show punched-out bone lesions, reminiscent of gout, and destruction of the joints. To help distinguish this arthropathy from rheumatoid arthritis, there is widening of the joint space and relatively little juxta-articular osteopenia in multicentric reticulohistiocytosis[(2)].

How is multicentric reticulohistiocytosis diagnosed?

The diagnosis is made by biopsy of skin or synovium. There is an infiltrate of large, multinucleated giant cells, and the cytoplasm has a ground glass appearance and stains with periodic acid-Schiff, probably for a glycolipid.

Concerning differential diagnoses, which diseases are most likely to be confused with multicentric reticulohistiocytosis?

With symmetrical polyarthritis, morning stiffness, nodules over the elbows, and joint erosions on radiography, rheumatoid arthritis is often mistakenly diagnosed and treated in a patient with multicentric reticulohistiocytosis. Differentiating features for multicentric reticulohistiocytosis are distal interphalangeal joint arthritis and the periungual distribution of cutaneous nodules. Another confounding type of arthritis, when there is prominent distal interphalangeal joint inflammation, is psoriatic arthritis. However, the skin lesions of multicentric reticulohistiocytosis are quite different than those of psoriasis, as described above [3].

How is this arthropathy treated?

Nonsteroidal antiinflammatory drugs and physical therapy are helpful in mild to moderate cases, but methotrexate or cyclophosphamide is warranted in intractable situations [4]. Use of the tumor necrosis factor-alpha antagonists for this syndrome is now being reported [5].

Is there an association of multicentric reticulohistiocytosis and malignancy?

Yes; about 25% of patients have an associated malignancy. Various malignancies have been associated [1]. Consequently, in some instances multicentric reticulohistiocytosis might be a paraneoplastic syndrome.

What is the prognosis of multicentric reticulohistiocytosis?

Progressive joint destruction occurs in approximately one-half of patients, with arthritis mutilans (opera-glass hands, or so-called "main en lorgnette") eventuating [3, 6]. Skin involvement can cause facial disfigurement.

KEY POINTS

- Multicentric reticulohistiocytosis is a peculiar dermatoarthritis characterized by the accumulation of lipid laden macrophages in the skin and joints.
- Skin nodules occur on the hands, elbows, face and ears.
- A characteristic coral bead appearance of these nodules on the nail beds should suggest the diagnosis.
- Severe involvement of the face can result in a leonine facies.
- Symmetric polyarthritis, with involvement of the distal interphalangeal joints, is the rule. The arthritis can be mutilating.

- A nonsteroidal antiinflammatory drug is effective in treating most cases, though in severe cases of MCR successful treatment requires methotrexate or cyclophosphamide.

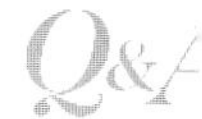

SECTION FIVE

CHAPTER 30

THERAPEUTICS

RELATIVELY SPECIFIC CYCLOOXYGENASE-2 INHIBITORS

John D Carter, Bryan A Bognar, Harold M Adelman

Why the need to invent a better mouse trap?

One of the primary mechanisms of action of the first generation nonsteroidal anti-inflammatory drugs (NSAIDs) is inhibition of both cyclooxygenase-1(COX-1) and cyclooxygenase-2 (COX-2). These enzymes catalyze the second reaction bringing arachidonic acid to the proinflammatory prostaglandins. COX-1 is a constitutive enzyme; that is, it is present in multiple tissues under normal circumstances. In fact, while COX1 helps form proinflammatory prostaglandins, it also exerts protective effects elsewhere, for instance the gastric mucosa and the kidneys, and fosters normal platelet function. Inhibition of these protective effects by the first generation NSAIDs leads to the toxicity of the COX-1 inhibitors, such as gastric and duodenal ulcers, nephropathy, and a bleeding diathesis. On the other hand, cyclooxygenase-2 is present primarily, but not exclusively, in areas of inflammation. It is probable, therefore, that inhibition primarily of COX-2 will help suppress inflammation with less GI toxicity than the first generation NSAIDs. The COX-2 inhibitors are not more potent than the COX-1 inhibitors, and renal toxicity is not less.

Which COX-2 inhibitors are available?

As of this writing, celecoxib and lumiracoxib are the only two COX- 2 agents available in the United States and the United Kingdom. Celecoxib's new black box warnings about cardiovascular and gastrointestinal side effects are to be heeded. In fact, all NSAIDs, prescription and over-the-counter, will have a warning about cardiovascular risks, see below.

Celecoxib is to be avoided in patients allergic to sulfonamides because of possible cross allergenicity, and also in patients with the triad of allergic rhinitis, nasal polyps and bronchospasm (Sampter's triad). Importantly, all NSAIDs are to be avoided in patients with Sampter's triad because of the risk of fatal bronchospasm. Lumiracoxib, a highly selective COX2 inhibitor, was approved in the UK by the Medicines and Healthcare products Regulatory Agency in September, 2003 for osteoarthritis. It is in common use in Europe and Latin America. Several studies, including the TARGET (Therapeutic Arthritis Research and Gastrointestinal Event Trial), have demonstrated an incidence of cardiovascular events comparable to ibuprofen and naproxen[105-107]. There was a question about the power of the study to exclude statistically significant differences in cardiovascular events, and about the exclusion from the study of patients with known and significant preexisting coronary artery disease[107,108]. Lumiracoxib showed a three to four-fold reduction in ulcer complications compared with non-steroidal anti-inflammatory drugs[105]. In the US, The Federal Drug Administration is presently studying lumiracoxib.

THE COX-2 QUANDARY – WHAT'S HAPPENING?

THE GOOD, THE BAD, THE UGLY

On September 30, 2004, one pharmaceutical company voluntarily recalled rofecoxib from the market worldwide because of data indicating an increased risk of heart attack and stroke, and in April 2005, another company withdrew valdecoxib for the same concern. Celecoxib will have a black box warning about this potential problem. Mechanistically, the relatively selective cyclooxygenase-2 (COX-2) inhibitors block the synthesis of thromboxane and prostacyclin. Thromboxane increases platelet aggregation and causes vasoconstriction, while prostacyclin reduces platelet aggregation and causes vasodilation. The relative degree to which this inhibition occurs might determine whether deleterious vascular thrombotic events happen.

THE GOOD: The relatively selective COX-2 inhibitors approximately halve the incidence of gastrointestinal ulcers compared with the first generation nonsteroidal anti-inflammatory drugs. Ulcers, hemorrhage, perforation, and obstruction lead to 76,000 hospitalizations and 7,600 deaths a year in the

United States[1]. Approximately 10% of patients hospitalized for an NSAID-induced upper GI hemorrhage die[2]. The relatively selective COX-2 inhibitors significantly decrease these complications.

THE BAD: In the APPROVe (Adenomatous Polyp Prevention on Vioxx) study, 2,600 people who had removal of colorectal polyps were randomly assigned to receive rofecoxib (NSAIDs are known to inhibit polyps) or placebo. Approximately 3.5% of those taking rofecoxib and 1.9% on placebo had a myocardial infarction or stroke during the trial as of the third year of the study, an excess of 16 events per 1000 patients[3]. In another study, the VIGOR trial, rofecoxib, and naproxen were compared in patients with arthritis[4]. Myocardial infarction and stroke occurred significantly more often in patients taking rofecoxib than naproxen, 46 vs 20 events among approximately 4000 patients in each group. The duration of treatment was a median of nine months[4]. Similarly, data indicate an increased risk of myocardial infarction and stroke for valdecoxib and for celecoxib at higher doses. The first-generation NSAIDs are associated with increased risk myocardial infarction and stroke as well.

THE UGLY: Patients with inflammatory arthropathies who rely on NSAIDs and who might now have to stop their NSAIDs are now facing a dilemma.

So what should we do?

For patients at high risk of gastrointestinal complications, such as prior gastrointestinal ulcer disease or bleeding, and with no known risks for cardiovascular disease, for whom an NSAID is clearly and strongly indicated, e.g., those with severe arthritis not responding to other measures, the relatively selective COX-2 inhibitor, celecoxib, with all due prudence, may be considered[5,6]. The dose of celecoxib should not exceed 200 mg daily. The foremost way to avoid NSAID gastropathy is to combine an NSAID with a proton pump inhibitor. In general, use the lowest dose of the NSAID for the shortest time possible. Further studies will be telling.

What other options are there to minimize the GI side effects of the first generation NSAIDS?

Acetaminophen is now the drug of choice for mild to moderate osteoarthritis. Non-acetylated salicylates, such as salsalate and magnesium choline salicylate, are relatively safe, with little gastrointestinal or renal toxicity. These medications have no antiplatelet effect. The proton pump inhibitors and misoprostol, a prostaglandin E analogue, also decrease the frequency of stomach and duodenal complications from NSAIDs.

What about recent caveats concerning NSAIDs interfering with the cardioprotective effect of aspirin?

Recent literature concerning the possible interference of ibuprofen with the cardioprotective effect of aspirin has appeared[7]. Whether other NSAIDs might have this effect is being studied.

METHOTREXATE

Where does methotrexate place in the hierarchy of disease modifying antirheumatic drugs?

Methotrexate (MTX) is currently the DMARD of first choice in rheumatoid arthritis because of its sustained efficacy and because its toxicity is usually manageable. MTX was first used for the treatment of rheumatoid arthritis (RA) and psoriasis in 1951[8]. Numerous studies have detailed the efficacy of MTX in the treatment of rheumatoid arthritis[9,10]. MTX is also used successfully in other rheumatic diseases.

How is MTX administered?

MTX can be given either orally or intramuscularly. In most situations, it is given in doses of 7.5 to 20 mg once a week. MTX is available in 2.5 mg tablets and 25 mg/cc vials.

What seems to be the primary mechanism of action of MTX as a disease modifying anti-rheumatic drug (DMARD)?

The mechanisms of action of MTX in the rheumatic disease are not entirely clear. MTX inhibits dihydrofolate reductase and other folate-dependent enzymes, including aminoimidazole carboxamide-ribonucleotide (AICAR) transformylase[11]. By inhibiting AICAR transformylase, MTX increases adenosine levels, and adenosine inhibits the inflammatory process by interfering with leukocyte function and some inflammatory cytokines[12]. MTX also has some immunosuppressive effects.

What are the indications for using methotrexate in the rheumatic diseases?

Methotrexate is most commonly used in the treatment of severe rheumatoid arthritis and psoriatic arthritis. Recalcitrant polymyositis/dermatomyositis and systemic lupus erythematosus can respond to methotrexate. Remission of vasculitis can be maintained by methotrexate.

How should patients on methotrexate be monitored?

The American College of Rheumatology offers the following guidelines for monitoring patients on methotrexate (MTX):

Before starting therapy:

- CBC, liver chemistries, serum creatinine, and hepatitis B and C serologies;
- Liver biopsy for those with elevated aminotransferases, a history of heavy alcohol use, or hepatitis.

While on therapy:

- Liver chemistries every one to two months;
- Liver biopsy during therapy if amino aminotransferases are elevated in five of nine or six of 12 determinations over a one year period, or for any drop in serum albumin.

Should a liver biopsy be done in patients taking long-term methotrexate?

The American College of Rheumatology recommends liver biopsy for patients taking MTX who have:

- aminotransferases elevated in five of nine or six of 12 determinations over one year;
- any drop in serum albumin.

Methotrexate may be more hepatotoxic in patients with psoriasis than in patients with rheumatoid arthritis. Therefore, for patients on MTX for psoriatic arthritis, liver biopsy is recommended after each cumulative dose of 1.5 to 2.0 grams.

How is methotrexate metabolized and excreted?

After administration, the parent compound methotrexate is metabolized into several metabolites, all of which are highly bound to albumin. These compounds are eliminated by excretion from the kidneys as well as in the bile. Consequently, methotrexate should be avoided in patients with renal insufficiency or impaired hepatic function. In addition, great caution should be exercised in patients at risk of renal or hepatic impairment, including those with a history of diabetes mellitus, or heavy alcohol use. Obese patients are at increased risk of liver toxicity from MTX.

What is the value of concomitant folic acid therapy for patients on methotrexate?

Methotrexate is an analog of folic acid and interferes with DNA synthesis by inhibiting the activity of the enzyme dihydrofolate reductase. This inhibition is the mechanism of many of the toxic effects of methotrexate, and it might differ from the main antirheumatic mechanism of action discussed above. As such, supplemental folic acid is used to combat some of the side effects of methotrexate, including nausea and ulcerations of the mouth. Folic acid is typically given in doses ranging from one to three mg a day. It is currently unclear if folic acid supplementation may slightly mitigate the therapeutic efficacy of MTX.

Can methotrexate be used with other antirheumatic agents?

Yes, and it often is, for patients with recalcitrant disease. Methotrexate is reasonably safe in combination with hydroxychloroquine, sulfasalazine [13] leflunomide, infliximab, etanercept, adalimumab , cyclosporine, and tacrolimus.

Is there a survival benefit with the use of MTX?

Yes there is. In a cohort study of 1,240 patients with rheumatoid arthritis, the hazard ratio for all cause mortality was 0.4 for the patients treated with MTX. The reduction in cardiovascular mortality was statistically significant [14]. Whether leflunomide, anakinra, and the tumor necrosis factor-alpha blockers offer similar protection is not yet certain.

HYDROXYCHLOROQUINE

How did anti-malarial drugs become "adopted" as anti-rheumatic agents?

The use of anti-malarial medication in the rheumatic diseases can be traced to the 1890s, when they were used for the cutaneous manifestations of systemic lupus erythematosus. In the 1950s, British physicians observed beneficial antirheumatic effects of anti-malarials in patients with malaria who also had rheumatoid arthritis (RA) or systemic lupus erythematosus (SLE)[15]. Originally, these observations were made on patients who had received malaria prophylaxis with quinacrine. Later chloroquine, and finally hydroxychloroquine were developed in order to decrease the toxicity of the drug. Presently, anti-malarials are used commonly to treat RA and SLE.

What is its mechanism of action of anti-malarials in the rheumatic diseases?

The precise mechanism of action of hydroxychloroquine is not known. However, there are several theories on how the drug works. Hydroxychloroquine has a high affinity for acidic environments because it is a weak base[16]. Hence the drug accumulates in the acidic lysosomes that are bound to cell membranes. Once inside the lysosomal vesicles, the drug is acidified and therefore unable to diffuse back across the cell membrane. Consequently, a large accumulation of the drug is created in the lysosomal system of lymphocytes, macrophages, and fibroblasts, where its anti-rheumatic effect is believed to occur. Alkalinization of the lysosome theoretically interferes with its functions, that is, the enzymatic hydrolysis of particulate matter, including defunct organelles, foreign bodies, or the cell itself. In addition, hydroxychloroquine may dampen or completely inhibit the antigen processing ability of monocytes and macrophages, which in turn, inhibits the response of lymphocytes to foreign antigens. Lastly, the release of interleukin-1 from monocytes and macrophages is inhibited by hydroxychloroquine, probably mediated through its effect on the lysosomal system[16].

What kind of practical prescribing tips can be offered to patients?

Hydroxychloroquine is rapidly absorbed from the gastrointestinal tract. Patients should be advised to take this medication with food for greater tolerability.

While slowing the rate of absorption, taking the drug with food does not affect the bioavailability of the drug[17]. There is a great degree of variance in the bioavailability of the drug from patient to patient, which might partially explain the difference in patient response. The adverse gastrointestinal effects of hydroxychloroquine include nausea, diarrhea, and abdominal cramps, usually tolerable if taken with food[18]. Patients should also be informed that the therapeutic response to hydroxychloroquine is delayed. They may not start to see any effect until one month of therapy has elapsed, and the full effects should not be expected until about six months of therapy.

The maximum recommended dose for hydroxychloroquine is 6 mg/kg a day, which is approximately equivalent to 400 mg a day[16]; however, if the patient is substantially large or small, this dose should be adjusted accordingly.

What is the half-life of hydroxychloroquine?

The half-life of this drug is long, about 40 days. This means that there will be a three to four month delay before steady-state concentrations are achieved.

What is the evidence that hydroxychloroquine works in the rheumatic diseases?

In 1962, the earliest controlled clinical trials with hydroxychloroquine were reported. These trials showed that patients with RA had decreased tender and swollen joint counts as well as decreased morning stiffness while on hydroxychloroquine[19]. More recent, placebo-controlled, double-blinded studies have shown that 60-80% of patients with RA treated with hydroxychloroquine demonstrated improvement in standard parameters including functional class, joint counts, pain, grip strength, morning stiffness, patient and observer's assessments, and erythrosedimentation rates (ESR)[16]. A small proportion of patient achieved complete remission.

Patients with SLE on hydroxychloroquine often require less corticosteroids to suppress their disease. An important study by Bykerk, et al., published in 1991 determined the long-term necessity of hydroxychloroquine. They found that patients who had been well-controlled on hydroxychloroquine had more flares of lupus after they withdrew hydroxychloroquine[20]. While it is unclear if the withdrawal of the drug actually caused the flare, or if the drug was responsible for maintaining a quiescent state of the disease, it is clear that patients should be maintained on long-term hydroxychloroquine if possible. There have also been studies that suggest that hydroxychloroquine is useful in the treatment of the arthralgias, myalgias, and lymphadenopathy in patients with primary Sjögren syndrome [21]. These patients had less episodes of parotid gland swelling while on hydroxychloroquine. However, there was no increase in the salivary or lacrimal gland flow rates demonstrated with the use of this medication. Another interesting rheumatologic use of hydroxychloroquine is for the cutaneous manifestations of dermatomyositis. The drug, however, has not shown any benefit on the myositis aspect of this disease.

What precautions should be taken when prescribing hydroxychloroquine?

If hydroxychloroquine is prescribed within the recommended dosage range of up to 6 mg/kg a day, it is a safe medication. The most feared adverse reaction to the drug is irreversible retinopathy. This reaction is most commonly seen with chloroquine and rarely with hydroxychloroquine. Patients may complain of difficulty reading and seeing, photophobia, visual field defects, light flashes and streaks, or scotomata. A retrospective study of 1500 patients on less than 7 mg/kg a day of hydroxychloroquine revealed no cases of retinopathy [22]. However, it is still recommended that patients have an ophthalmological examination every six to twelve months for hydroxychloroquine retinopathy.

Approximately 3-5% of patients taking hydroxychloroquine may develop maculopapular rashes, or a variety of other skin eruptions. Also, this drug can rarely cause increased mucosal and skin pigmentation, with the latter being accentuated in dark-skinned individuals. Patients should be informed of this possible side effect.

The use of hydroxychloroquine in patients with psoriasis and porphyria may precipitate attacks. Therefore, the drug should be used with great caution in these patients. It should also be used with caution in patients with liver disease, alcoholism, or taking other known hepatotoxic drugs. Lastly, hydroxychloroquine should be avoided in patients that are pregnant or interested in becoming pregnant.

Are there any drug interactions with hydroxychloroquine?

There are no major drug interactions. However, calcium channel blockers, such as verapamil or diltiazem have been shown to increase blood levels of hydroxychloroquine. Patients on these drugs should be monitored for any increased toxicity of hydroxychloroquine. Hydroxychloroquine can be used safely in combination with corticosteroids, NSAIDs or other DMARDs.

What are the starting and maintenance doses of hydroxychloroquine?

Patients with RA are started on 400 to 600 mg daily, taken with a meal or glass of milk. When a response is observed, usually four to six weeks, the dose is decreased to 400 mg daily. If possible, a maintenance dose of 200 mg daily is advisable. The usual starting dose for patients with SLE is 400 mg once or twice daily. After there is sufficient response, the dose can be decreased to 200 to 400 mg daily.

SULFASALAZINE

What is sulfasalazine?

Sulfasalazine comprises the sulfonamide sulfapyridine and 5-aminosalicylate (5-ASA). Counter intuitively, it seems to be the sulfapyridine moiety and the complete sulfasalazine molecule that are active in rheumatoid arthritis and not 5-ASA. The latter is the active moiety in inflammatory bowel disease.

How did sulfasalazine "return" to rheumatology?

The sulfasalazine story is quite interesting. Of the disease modifying antirheumatic drugs (DMARDs), only sulfasalazine was originally intended for rheumatoid arthritis. Professor Nana Svartz of Stockholm is the pioneer in sulfasalazine use for rheumatoid arthritis [23]. Rheumatologists have "borrowed" the other DMARDs, such as methotrexate, hydroxychloroquine, gold and D-penicillamine, from other disciplines in medicine. Sulfasalazine was abandoned in the late 1940s for apparent lack of efficacy, to be rediscovered in the 1970s [24, 25]. European rheumatologists have used it for over 30 years. Presently, this medication is in common use in rheumatology worldwide, by itself and as part of combination regimens [26, 27, 28].

Who is a candidate for sulfasalazine?

This medication is intended for patients with moderate, active rheumatoid arthritis. It is used with a nonsteroidal antiinflammatory drug or in combination with other DMARDs. Sulfasalazine can also be helpful for some patients with the arthritis of inflammatory bowel disease. This drug is also useful for patients with the chronic form of post-dysentery reactive arthritis and in the spondyloarthritides[29, 30].

How does this medication work?

The mechanism of action of sulfasalazine is not clear. The intact sulfasalazine molecule inhibits nuclear factor kappa B, as do glucocorticoids, and thereby inhibits transcription of central mediators of the immune response. In addition, this drug also induces apoptosis of macrophages. Sulfasalazine is split into sulfapyridine and 5-ASA in the colon by the enzyme azoreductase, produced by coliform bacteria. The antimicrobial effect of sulfapyridine is unlikely to be relevant in rheumatoid arthritis.

How is this medication administered?

Sulfasalazine is given orally and the dose should be increased gradually for better tolerance. Start with 500 mg once a day, and increase by 500 mg daily at weekly intervals to a maximum of two grams daily. If the response is not satisfactory, and the patient is tolerating the drug well, the dose can be further increased to a maximum of three grams daily, in divided doses. If mild toxicity occurs, the dose can be decreased to 1.5 g daily or 1 gram daily.

What is the evidence for efficacy?

A meta-analysis published by M.E. Weinblatt and colleagues in 1999 of eight placebo controlled, randomized trials, which included 552 patients receiving sulfasalazine and 351 patients on placebo, reported that treatment was significantly more effective than placebo[31]. Specifically, morning stiffness, the number of painful joints, the number of swollen joints, and joint pain were significantly improved with sulfasalazine compared with placebo. The erythrosedimentation rate and C-reactive protein were decreased as well.

What are the side effects and toxicity of sulfasalazine?

Most patients can take sulfasalazine without significant problems. No major drug interactions have been reported. The significant side effects are:

- Hematologic, with early (within the first three months) agranulocytosis, or aplastic anemia, hemolytic anemia, and megaloblastic anemia by causing folate deficiency;

- Rash;
- Hepatitis;
- Gastrointestinal intolerance with nausea, vomiting and diarrhea;
- Headache or dizziness, severe enough to require discontinuation;
- Fever;
- Oligospermia, reversible on discontinuation of the drug.

Slow initiation of therapy and serial monitoring of laboratory tests can lessen the significance of the side effects. A complete blood count and liver enzymes should be performed at the initiation of therapy and every two weeks for the first three months (when agranulocytosis occurs, it usually does so in the first three months), then monthly for the second three months, and every three months thereafter [32].

What are the contraindications of sulfasalazine?

Sulfasalazine is contraindicated in patients with allergies to sulfa drugs or salicylates, or patients with porphyria, gastrointestinal or urinary obstruction, and children under two years of age. Sulfasalazine is to be used with caution if at all in patients with glucose-6-phosphate dehydrogenase deficiency, or renal or hepatic function impairment.

Tetracycline Derivatives

The tetracycline derivatives minocycline and doxycycline have antiinflammatory and immune modulatory effects apart from their antibiotic activity [33, 34]. They inactivate matrix metalloproteinase activity, such as that of collagenase and gelatinase, enzymes that degrade articular cartilage. They also have an immune modulatory effect on T-cell and neutrophil function. Minocycline and doxycycline are being used with a modicum of success in early rheumatoid arthritis and osteoarthritis – see their respective sections [35, 36]. In rheumatoid arthritis, doxycycline should be used with methotrexate for efficacy.

LEFLUNOMIDE

What is the mechanism of action of leflunomide?

Leflunomide works by inhibiting the de novo synthesis of pyrimidine by interfering with dihydroorotate dehydrogenase, an enzyme involved in its synthesis [37]. By this mechanism, leflunomide has antiproliferative and antiinflammatory properties.

What is the active form of leflunomide?

The active form of leflunomide is a metabolite that is formed after oral administration of the drug. It is unclear where the drug is actually metabolized, but it is thought to occur primarily in the gastrointestinal tract and liver. Leflunomide is broken down into one main metabolite, A77 1726, also referred to as M1, and many other minor metabolites. The active metabolite, M1, is responsible for virtually all of its activity in vivo [37].

What is the drug's half-life?

The drug has a long half-life, estimated to be approximately two weeks. The recommended dose is 20 mg daily, without a loading dose formally used in the United States. There are less GI side effects without using a loading dose [38] [5].

How is leflunomide eliminated from the body?

The drug is primarily eliminated through the kidneys and by direct biliary excretion. In the first 96 hours, leflunomide is primarily excreted by the kidneys; fecal elimination tends to predominate after that point. It has been demonstrated that approximately 43% is eliminated in the urine and 48% in the feces. The small remainder of the drug is metabolized in other parts of the body.

Can patients with renal or hepatic insufficiency take this medication?

The answer to this question is unclear. Leflunomide was studied in only six patients with renal failure requiring either continuous ambulatory peritoneal dialysis (CAPD) or hemodialysis. None of these six patients had increased levels of the active metabolite (M1); however, the free fraction of M1 was almost twice that seen in patients with normal renal function. The reason is unclear. None of the six patients had toxic side effects from leflunomide. However, given the small number of patients studied, and the abnormal free fraction of the drug, leflunomide should be administered to patients with renal insufficiency with great caution if at all. Given the fact that the liver and biliary system seem to play a crucial role in the metabolism of the drug, and the possibility of hepatotoxicity from leflunomide itself, this drug should not be given to patients with hepatic insufficiency.

Are there any significant drug interactions with leflunomide?

Leflunomide has been shown to increase the free fraction of certain NSAIDs, especially diclofenac and ibuprofen. In vitro studies indicate that the active metabolite, M1, inhibits cytochrome P450 2C9, which is responsible for the metabolism of many NSAIDs[39]. This point should be kept in mind when prescribing a combination of leflunomide and NSAIDs, especially diclofenac and ibuprofen. There is no specific drug-drug interaction between leflunomide and methotrexate. However, the combination does lead to increased hepatotoxicity, so provider beware. Two other leflunomide interactions worth noting concern rifampin and tolbutamide: rifampin increases the peak levels of M1 by approximately 40%, and M1 tends to increase the free fraction of tolbutamide by about 13-50%. Both of these combinations should be used with caution. Lastly, the coadministration of leflunomide and cholestyramine results in a rapid and significant decrease in the active metabolite of leflunomide, M1. This interaction will be discussed in more detail later in this chapter.

What is the indication for leflunomide?

Leflunomide has been proven to be efficacious for the treatment of rheumatoid arthritis (RA) in three controlled trials. The first trial randomized 482 patients with active rheumatoid arthritis to receive six months of therapy with either leflunomide, 20 mg a day after a 100 mg loading dose for each of three days, methotrexate, 7.5 mg per week increasing to 15 mg per week if necessary, or placebo[39]. All of the patients in this study received folic acid 1 mg twice daily. The second trial compared leflunomide (the same dosing), sulfasalazine (two grams daily), or placebo in 358 subjects with RA[39]. The final study compared 999 patients with active RA with the same dose of leflunomide as in the previous studies, vs. methotrexate[39]. Folate supplementation was used in only 10% of the patients. These three trials revealed that there were no consistent differences between leflunomide and methotrexate, or leflunomide and sulfasalazine. The effect of leflunomide is usually evident by one month, maximizes by three to six months, and continues throughout the use of the drug. Accordingly, leflunomide has been shown to improve both subjective and objective measures of RA, including retarding new joint erosions and joint space narrowing[40,41]. It does not, however, appear to be superior to methotrexate or sulfasalazine[42, 43].

What special precautions should be taken when prescribing leflunomide?

Leflunomide can be hepatotoxic. Treatment with this drug has been associated with increases in liver aminotransferases. Most elevations are mild (less than or equal to two-fold the upper limit of normal) and they tend to resolve even with continued therapy. More pronounced elevations in liver aminotransferases (greater than three times the upper limit of normal) usually require dose reduction (to 10 mg daily) or discontinuation of the drug. For this reason, liver aminotransferases should be checked prior to initiating therapy, at monthly intervals initially, and then periodically depending on the clinical setting.
It may be prudent to obtain a hepatitis profile prior to beginning therapy with this drug. Pregnancy should be excluded prior to starting a patient on leflunomide, and the drug is contraindicated in pregnant women or in women considering pregnancy. Leflunomide is teratogenic in rats, causing anophthalmia, microphthalmia, and internal hydrocephalus[44]. It also causes an increase in embryo loss. In addition, mothers who are breastfeeding should not use this drug. Studies on males were not performed; thus, men wishing to father a child should not take leflunomide. It is also important to remember that leflunomide is an immunosuppressive agent. Although there was no reported increased incidence of infections, malignancies, or lymphoproliferative disorders, long-term studies need to be performed to exclude this possibility. The combination of leflunomide with TNF-inhibiting drugs is not well studied, and for that reason it is not currently recommended. Finally, it must be kept in mind that leflunomide has a very long half-life. If a patient is considering pregnancy, or the use of a live vaccine, it is easy to forget that they were taking leflunomide in the recent past.

Is there any way to eliminate the drug more quickly considering its long half-life?

There is a way to eliminate the drug more quickly if patients show signs of toxicity, or if they desire pregnancy, even after stopping the medication. The administration of 8 grams of cholestyramine three times daily for 11 days has been shown to decrease plasma levels to undetectable. Plasma levels, however, should be verified by two separate tests at least 14 days apart. Without using cholestyramine, it may take as long as two years to reach undetectable levels.

What is the proper dosage and administration of leflunomide?

The previously used loading dose causes nausea, diarrhea, and abdominal cramps therefore patients are now started on 20 mg daily. If the 20 mg dose is not tolerated, leflunomide may be decreased to 10 mg daily. Patients should be observed carefully after dose reductions, as it may take several weeks for drug levels to decline.

COMBINATION DISEASE MODIFYING ANTI-RHEUMATIC DRUG (DMARD) THERAPY

A major shift in paradigm among rheumatologists in the last 15 years is the *early* (within *three* months) use of combination DMARDs for patients with moderately severe, *active* rheumatoid arthritis. This concept is now so important that we devote a separate section to it, despite already having discussed it several times in this book.

Why is institution of early combination DMARD therapy considered such a good idea now?

Rheumatoid arthritis involves a multiplicity of pathogenic mechanisms, and combination DMARD therapy has a higher chance of effectiveness. Furthermore, combination therapy permits the use of lower doses of each medication and might result in less toxicity. A variety of combinations have been evaluated. In addition, severe rheumatoid arthritis is now recognized as a potentially lethal disease. On average, women lose approximately ten years of life and men four years. Causes of death in rheumatoid arthritis include infection, lymphoma, cervical spine disease, amyloidosis, interstitial pulmonary fibrosis, vasculitis, coronary heart disease, and medication side effects. Consequently, "treat patients before there are joint erosions" is the current battle cry.

What are the markers portending severe, progressive rheumatoid arthritis?

Once considered too toxic, early combination DMARD therapy is now deemed appropriate for rheumatoid patients with markers of severe, progressive disease. Such ominous markers include unremitting synovitis despite maximum NSAID therapy, multiple joint involvement early in the course, high titer rheumatoid factor (≥1:640), the presence of rheumatoid nodules, and other extraarticular manifestations of rheumatoid arthritis, such as vasculitis or scleritis. The modified Health Assessment Questionnaire, filled out by the patient, is a very good prognosticator of threat to life by rheumatoid arthritis.

What are some DMARD combinations used by rheumatologists?

Daniel McCarty and his group at the Medical College of Wisconsin in Milwaukee were the pioneers in combination DMARD therapy in the 1980s. Their seminal paper in JAMA on cyclophosphamide, azathioprine and, hydroxychloroquine led the way to further studies of combination therapy for intractable rheumatoid arthritis. The group subsequently decided to replace cyclophosphamide with methotrexate to lower the regimen's risk of causing cancer. Currently, methotrexate is the linchpin of combination DMARD therapy. The combinations most used now are methotrexate, hydroxychloroquine, and sulfasalazine. O'Dell and colleagues prospective, randomized controlled study published in Arthritis & Rheumatism in 2002 showed a 67% remission rate, and side effects no greater than for single DMARD therapy. Among other combinations that are being studied and used are methotrexate – sulfasalazine; methotrexate - hydroxychloroquine; methotrexate – leflunomide; and methotrexate - biologic agents [(46-53)]. A very aggressive regimen up front consists of prednisone, 60 mg daily tapered to 10 mg daily over five weeks, with methotrexate and sulfasalazine. This effective approach, from the Netherlands, is the so-called COBRA regimen - for *Combinatietherapie Bij Reumatoide Artritis* - and is popular among some rheumatologists [(54)]. Toxicity is still being evaluated.

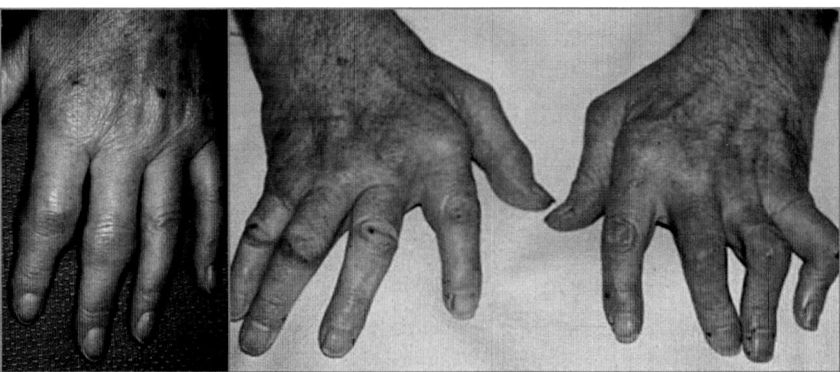

Figure 1. *Left Panel: Early rheumatoid arthritis of the hand.*
Reproduced with kind permission of the American College of Rheumatology.

Right panel: Late, destructive rheumatoid arthritis of the hand. With modern therapy such as the tumor necrosis factor alpha blockers, prevention of progression of RA from early changes can be achieved.
Wright G, Musgrave Park Hospital, Belfast, Northern Ireland.

What does the future hold?

Molecular biology, genomics and gene therapy of the autoimmune diseases hold great promise; the future is exciting.

THE BIOLOGICAL ANTIRHEUMATIC AGENTS

What is tumor necrosis factor-alpha?

Tumor necrosis factor-alpha (TNF-alpha) is a peptide that mediates inflammation and tissue damage through its two cell membrane receptors. TNF-alpha is synthesized mainly by macrophages responding to inflammatory stimuli.

What are the available tumor necrosis factor alpha blockers?

The three tumor necrosis factor alpha blockers available at this time are etanercept, infliximab and adalimumab.

ETANERCEPT

What is etanercept, and how does it work?

Etanercept is a *soluble* tumor necrosis factor-alpha *receptor*. It is a genetically engineered fusion protein, consisting of two identical chains to the extracellular ligand-binding portion of the human 75kd tumor necrosis factor receptor (TNFR) linked to the Fc portion of human IgG1. Etanercept "sops up" and inactivates tumor necrosis factor-alpha (TNF-alpha) by preventing its interaction with the cell surface receptors. It also inhibits human lymphotoxin [55-57]. TNF plays an important role in the inflammatory pathogenesis of rheumatoid arthritis. It regulates leukocyte migration and induces certain other proinflammatory cytokines, such as interleukin-6. Elevated levels of TNF are found in the synovial fluid of patients with rheumatoid arthritis. This cytokine also increases synovial fluid levels of metalloproteinase-3, an important enzyme in the destructive milieu of the rheumatoid synovia.

How is etanercept administered?

Etanercept must be administered either intravenously or subcutaneously. There is no oral form of the drug. Most often the drug is given subcutaneously, and the patient can be taught to self-administer it at home. Sites for self-injection include the thigh, abdomen, and upper arm, and it is suggested to rotate injection sites. The medication is supplied in single use vials and is reconstituted in one ml of sterile, bacteriostatic water. Etanercept usually reaches maximum serum concentrations approximately 72 hours after it is administered subcutaneously, and it has a half-life of 115 hours. Consequently, etanercept should be administered twice weekly. Recently a prefilled 50 mg vial of etanercept was made available, administered weekly.

What is the efficacy of etanercept?

Etanercept was approved in November of 1998 by the FDA for the treatment of patients with moderate to severe, active rheumatoid arthritis (RA) who have not responded adequately to one or more other disease modifying agents. The efficacy of etanercept has been well-established in clinical trials of patients with severe, active RA. These patients demonstrated decreased disease activity, increased functional activity, and improved health-related quality of life. These improvements have been shown to be sustained in studies as long as five years, and the studies are ongoing. In a recent, randomized, double-blinded, placebo-controlled trial with blinded joint assessors, there was a 20% American College of Rheumatology (ACR) response in 59% of the etanercept-treated group, versus 11% in the placebo group at six months of treatment (58). Also, a 50% ACR response was shown in 40% of the etanercept group versus 5% of the placebo group. Lastly, significantly more etanercept treated patients achieved a 70% ACR response (58). Consequently, etanercept seems to be quite effective in the treatment of moderate to severe rheumatoid arthritis. There are also recent trials that have proven the efficacy of etanercept in other types of inflammatory arthritis including psoriatic arthritis and ankylosing spondylitis (59, 60). This drug is now FDA indicated for the treatment of both psoriatic arthritis and ankylosing spondylitis.

How well does etanercept prevent radiographic progression of rheumatoid arthritis?

Recent data shows that etanercept in combination with methotrexate does very well at slowing, or perhaps even halting, the radiographic progression of rheumatoid arthritis. When etanercept is compared to methotrexate at two years of therapy the total Sharp score (a composite radiographic score consisting of joint erosions and joint space narrowing) improved to a significant degree (61).

How quickly does etanercept work and what happens if it is discontinued?

Clinical response to etanercept is usually quite rapid, beginning as early as two weeks after the initiation of therapy. Approximately 50% of patients who are going to respond to etanercept will do so by two weeks. Improvement at two weeks of therapy included such areas as arthritis specific health status, vitality, and mental and general health parameters. Studies have also shown that if etanercept therapy is discontinued, pre-treatment symptoms return. Consequently, the beneficial effects of the medication require continued therapy.

What are the main adverse reactions and side effects of etanercept?

Etanercept is generally well tolerated. Patients with rheumatoid arthritis treated in controlled trials, serious adverse events occurred in four per cent of subjects treated with etanercept, versus five per cent with placebo-treated patients [62]. The most common adverse reaction encountered with etanercept is a local injection site reaction that does occur in a statistically significantly higher proportion of treated patients than those given placebo injections. The local reactions were mild to moderate, and they included erythema, pruritus, pain, or swelling. These reactions were usually mild enough that they did not require discontinuation of the drug.

Also, it is important to bear in mind that etanercept is an immuno-suppressive agent. There is a slight increase in the rate of infections in patients receiving etanercept, upper respiratory infections and sinusitis being the most frequent. Although, there has been no conclusive evidence of an increase in the incidence of serious infections, etanercept should not be initiated in a patient with an active infection, and the drug should be stopped if a patient taking etanercept develops an infection. Lastly, the rate of malignancies has not been increased in the current trials, however longer studies are needed. There has been a recent question raised about the possibility of increased rates of lymphomas in patients taking TNF-inhibiting drugs [63]. While some of this data comes from clinical trials, the majority of it relies on post-marketing reporting. These early data seems to suggest that the small increased risk for lymphoma seen in patients taking TNF-inhibiting drugs is in keeping with the small increased risk of lymphoma known to exist in patients with rheumatoid arthritis. However, there is not yet a definitive answer to this question, and further data are needed.

Does etanercept induce antibodies to itself or induce autoantibodies?

Etanercept is a genetically engineered TNFR, so theoretically it could generate an immune response to itself. Patients have been tested at multiple times during the course of therapy for the presence of antibodies to etanercept. Antibodies were detected at least once in 16% of the patients. However, their clinical response to the drug did not wane nor were there increased adverse reactions [62]. Consequently, while antibodies to etanercept periodically may be produced, they do not seem to have any clinical significance. Treatment with etanercept has been associated with the formation of some autoantibodies. There was a slight increase in the number of patients that developed ANAs (11% versus 5% for placebo) and anti-double stranded DNA antibodies (15% versus 4% for placebo) [62]. However, none of these patients developed lupus symptoms or any new autoimmune diseases.

Can etanercept be used in combination with DMARDs?

Etanercept has been well studied in combination with methotrexate. One study, a 24-week, randomized, double-blinded trial compared the combination of etanercept with methotrexate, and methotrexate with placebo. This study concluded that the combination of etanercept with methotrexate provided additional clinical benefit to methotrexate alone, and that there was no increased toxicity with the combination of the two drugs. At 24 weeks, 71% of the etanercept/methotrexate combination patients versus 27% of the methotrexate/ placebo patients met the ACR 20 criteria of improvement. As for the percentage of patients meeting the ACR 50 criteria, 39% of the etanercept/ methotrexate combination patients versus only three percent of the methotrexate and placebo patients achieved this goal [64]. Consequently, there is a clear benefit in the combination of these two DMARDs in patients with severe rheumatoid arthritis, and there seems to be no increased toxicity. This combination holds promise for the treatment of patients with previously recalcitrant rheumatoid arthritis. There needs to be studies of this combination in other types of severe arthritis. Patients on leflunomide and methotrexate are at a greater risk of bone marrow toxicity and this side effect must be closely monitored [65].

Can pregnant women or women wishing to become pregnant take etanercept?

Unfortunately, there are no studies of etanercept in pregnant women. The drug is currently rated a pregnancy category B, which means it is presumed to be safe only by animal studies. However it is important to remember that animal data does not always mirror human response, and there have been reports of birth defects in women on etanercept [66, 67]. Further data are needed.

Can etanercept be used with other nonDMARD medications for rheumatoid arthritis?

There have been no drug interactions reported with the use of etanercept. NSAIDs, salicylates, glucocorticoids, and methotrexate can be administered safely in combination with etanercept.

What is the proper dose of etanercept?

Three doses of etanercept have been studied, a 10 and 25 mg dose given subcutaneously twice weekly, and 50 mg weekly. The 25 mg dose has shown clear clinical benefit, without any increased toxicity. Consequently, 25 mg subcutaneously twice weekly, or 50 mg weekly, is the recommended dose for patients with moderate to severe rheumatoid arthritis.

INFLIXIMAB

What is infliximab and how does it work?

Another tumor necrosis factor-alpha blocker, infliximab is a chimeric monoclonal antibody against this cytokine. A chimera is a structure consisting of diverse genetic constitution. Infliximab is composed of 75% human proteins and 25% mouse proteins. It binds to both circulating and cell membrane-bound tumor necrosis factor alpha.

How is infliximab administered?

Infliximab is administered by intravenous infusion. It is given once every eight weeks for the chronic treatment of rheumatoid arthritis; however, the initial doses are more frequent. The recommended protocol for the administration of infliximab consists of treatment at zero, two, and six weeks, then every eight weeks thereafter. It has only been studied in combination with methotrexate in the treatment of rheumatoid arthritis, so it is recommended that methotrexate be co-administered with this drug when treating rheumatoid arthritis.

What is the half-life of infliximab?

The half-life of infliximab is eight to ten days. The co-administration of methotrexate prolongs the half-life of this medication.

What is infliximab approved for and how efficacious is it?

Infliximab is approved for the treatment of rheumatoid arthritis, Crohn's disease, psoriatic arthritis and ankylosing spondylitis. Trials have demonstrated clear benefit with this medication in the treatment of all of these conditions. The largest trial to establish the efficacy of infliximab in the treatment of rheumatoid arthritis was the ATTRACT Trial [(68)]. This 102-week trial clearly established the efficacy of this drug. At 30 weeks of therapy, patients who were treated with 3 mg/kg of infliximab every eight weeks (in combination with methotrexate) achieved ACR 20, 50, and 70 scores of 50%, 27%, and 8% respectively. The scores at 102 weeks were very similar, thus, its efficacy is sustained. The vitality scores were also significantly improved with this same dose at both 54 and 102 weeks. This medication was also studied at three other doses (3 mg/kg every four weeks, 10 mg/kg every eight weeks, and 10 mg/kg every four weeks). The ACR scores were slightly better at the higher doses. The current recommended starting dose is 3 mg/kg every eight weeks, but this drug dose allow flexible dosing. It is important to remember that dose adjustment can substantially increase the cost.

Does infliximab affect the radiographic progression of rheumatoid arthritis?

Yes. This drug has been shown to do quite well at retarding radiographic progression, perhaps even stopping it altogether, with background methotrexate. In the ATTRACT Trial, the mean change in the Total Sharp Score was seven versus 1.3 when comparing methotrexate and infliximab with methotrexate respectively at 54 weeks of therapy (p value < 0.001).

How quickly does infliximab work?

Similar to the other TNF-inhibiting drugs, infliximab often works as soon as two weeks of therapy. In the ATTRACT Trial, almost 70% of the patients who were going to respond to the drug did so at two weeks of therapy. It is, however, important to note that some patients may take a couple of months before a response is seen.

What are the main side effects of infliximab?

Generally, infliximab is well tolerated. However, there is the possibility of both infusion reactions and long-term complications. Infusion reactions, if present, are generally mild. They consist of headaches, nausea, and light-headedness. More serious infusion reactions including hypotension, chest pain, and anaphylaxis have been reported, but thankfully are very rare.

Long- term complications include a slight increased risk for serious infections, including opportunistic infections. Early data from the trials revealed a slight increase risk for patients developing tuberculosis while on infliximab [(69)]. TNF alpha is instrumental in granuloma formation, so it was felt that this was re-activation of latent tuberculosis. A subsequent recommendation was made that all patients be screened with a purified protein derivative (PPD) skin test, and perhaps a screening chest X-ray, prior to instituting infliximab. If either are positive, infliximab is contraindicated. If this recommendation is followed, the chance of reactivating tuberculosis after starting infliximab is virtually non-existent. There is, however, emerging data that suggests that patients who are PPD positive can be treated with isoniazid for nine months in order to use infliximab safely (or the other TNF-inhibitors) [(70)]. Whether or not you must withhold infliximab until the nine months of antituberculous therapy is completed, or infliximab can be safely instituted at some point during the nine months of therapy, is not clearly defined.

Another relative contraindication to the use of infliximab (as well as the other TNF-inhibitors) is the presence of underlying moderate to severe congestive heart failure. A recent concern with infliximab (and other TNF-inhibiting drugs) is the possible slight increase risk for lymphoma [(70)]. The current feeling is that the slight increase incidence of lymphoma in patients on these drugs is compatible with the increased risk for lymphoma from their underlying rheumatoid arthritis. However, more data are needed to definitively address this concern.

Does the fact that this medication contains 25% mouse proteins pose any unique problems?

The answer to this is not really clear. There is autoantibody formation to the drug but it does not seem to be out of line with the other TNF-inhibiting drugs. However, it is important to keep in mind that this drug has only been well studied in combination with methotrexate in the setting of rheumatoid arthritis, whereas the other anti-TNF drugs do have monotherapy trials. Theoretically, the co-administration of methotrexate could decrease the autoantibody formation. The absence of infliximab monotherapy trials in the treatment of RA precludes us from answering this question. While there have been cases of "lupus-like" syndromes, there does not appear to be a strong correlation with autoantibody formation. The majority of patients who develop autoantibodies have no apparent change in their clinical condition.

ADALIMUMAB

What is adalimumab and how does it work?

Adalimumab is a fully human recombinant monoclonal antibody against TNF-alpha. It works by binding to, and thereby inhibiting, both circulating and cell-membrane bound TNF-alpha. By inhibiting TNF-alpha, this medication blocks the inflammatory cascade that TNF-alpha causes in rheumatoid arthritis and other inflammatory conditions.

What diseases can adalimumab treat?

The FDA approved adalimumab in December of 2002 for the treatment of moderate to severe rheumatoid arthritis. It is indicated to decrease the signs and symptoms and inhibit the structural damage of rheumatoid arthritis. It can be used either as monotherapy or in combination with other DMARD's (in particular methotrexate). Adalimumab is also an approved treatment for psoriatic arthritis, and it is being studied in the treatment of ankylosing spondylitis and inflammatory bowel disease.

How is adalimumab administered?

Adalimumab comes in pre-filled syringes and is self-injected subcutaneously. Its current recommended dose for rheumatoid arthritis is 40 mg once every two weeks. The half-life of the drug is approximately 14 days.

How efficacious is adalimumab in the treatment of rheumatoid arthritis?

Adalimumab works quite well in the treatment of rheumatoid arthritis. There have been three pivotal trials in assessing adalimumab[72-74]. Two of these trials studied adalimumab in combination with methotrexate (ARMADA and DE019) and one assessed adalimumab monotherapy (DE011). All of these trials show that adalimumab consistently decreases the signs and symptoms of RA as well as inhibits the structural damage. In DE019, the ACR 20, 50, and 70 scores were 63%, 39%, and 21% respectively at 24 weeks of therapy. In DE011 (monotherapy trial), the ACR scores were 46%, 22%, and 12% respectively. Another, perhaps more accurate, method to assess therapeutic efficacy in RA trials is the DAS28 (Disease Activity Severity) score. This score represents a composite of the swollen/tender joint counts, sedimentation rate, and general health assessment. Adalimumab statistically significantly improved the DAS28 score in all three aforementioned trials at six months of therapy.

Can adalimumab improve disability in rheumatoid arthritis patients?

The Health Assessment Questionnaire (HAQ) is a frequently used tool to assess functional disability in RA trials. It is generally accepted that a decrease of 0.22 points or more in the HAQ score represents significant improvement. The HAQ score decreased by 0.58 and 0.56 points in the ARMADA and DE019 trials respectively at six months of therapy. The HAQ score decreased by 0.38 at six months in DE011 (monotherapy).

Does adalimumab improve the constitutional symptoms associated with rheumatoid arthritis?

There was significant improvement in the vitality scores in all three of the aforementioned trials. Fatigue scores were shown to significantly improve in both the ARMADA and DE019 trials.

Does adalimumab affect the radiographic progression of rheumatoid arthritis?

Yes. The decrease in structural damage seen in the adalimumab trials is quite impressive. At 52 weeks of therapy in the DE019 trial (methotrexate/placebo versus methotrexate/adalimumab), the Total Sharp Score was 2.7 versus 0.1 (p value < 0.001). The joint erosion score and joint space narrowing score were 1.7 and 1.1 versus 0 and 0 respectively (p value < 0.001 for both).

How quickly does adalimumab work?

Similar to the other TNF-inhibiting drugs, results can be expected as soon as two weeks. Similar to infliximab, approximately 70% who are going to respond to adalimumab do so within two weeks.

Since this drug is "fully human", can you develop autoantibodies to adalimumab?

Yes. Although, this drug is a recombinant fully human antibody, approximately 12% of patients develop antibodies to the drug. While it has been speculated that those patients who develop autoantibodies to the drug demonstrate decreased clinical response, this is not definitively proven.

What are the potential side effects of adalimumab?

In the clinical trials, there were 2,468 patients who received adalimumab. Overall, the adverse events were the same as placebo with the infection rate similar to placebo also. However, serious infections were increased when compared to placebo [75]. There were thirteen cases of tuberculosis in the clinical trials. Similar to the recommendation with infliximab, it is recommended that you screen patients with a PPD, and perhaps a chest X-ray, prior to instituting adalimumab. Lastly, there were 10 cases of lymphoma in the clinical trials in the patients who received adalimumab. This equates to a standardized incidence ratio (SIR) of 5.4. The SIR of lymphoma in patients with RA has been reported to range from 2-26 in previous trials. Thus, the SIR of lymphoma in adalimumab treated- patients fall well within the range of RA patients in general. However, there were no cases of lymphoma in the placebo groups of the adalimumab trials. As with the other TNF-inhibiting drugs, more data are needed to determine if there is, indeed, a small increased risk of lymphoma with this drug.

TNF- alpha Blockers– Summary

Marked progress is being made in the treatment of rheumatoid arthritis. Used early, within three months of diagnosis, in severe active RA, the TNF-alpha blockers have proven to change the course of the disease [76, 77].

Are there any differences between the three TNF-inhibiting drugs currently available?

While these three drugs are generally similar in their biologic target, there are subtle differences. The lack of head to head trials makes it impossible to determine if there are subtle differences regarding efficacy in the treatment of rheumatoid arthritis with these three drugs. However, the most obvious difference between these three drugs is that two of them are antibodies (infliximab and adalimumab) and one is a receptor (etanercept). Infliximab has been shown to be cytolytic in vitro against the cell that produces TNF, whereas etanercept is not. Whether or not this difference has any clinical or adverse event implications is not clear. However, this may explain why infliximab has been proven to work in Crohn's disease and etanercept did not. This therapeutic difference is not appreciated in the treatment of rheumatoid arthritis.

It is also very difficult to ascertain whether some of the current concerns with these drugs represent a class effect or if there is truly variation among the individual drugs. This debate primarily revolves around the incidence of opportunistic infections (primarily tuberculosis, histoplasmosis, and Listeria) and the possible increased risk of lymphoma. More data are needed to address these important concerns.

ANAKINRA

What is the biologic target of anakinra?

Anakinra targets the receptor for the cytokine interleukin 1 (IL-1). Among many other effects, IL-1 mediates cartilage destruction by stimulating the production of collagenase (matrix metalloproteinase-1) and stromelysin.

What is the evidence of efficacy?

A recombinant human interleukin 1 receptor antagonist, (IL-1ra), anakinra is modestly effective in controlling moderate to severe, active rheumatoid arthritis. Using ACR-20 criteria, studies show improvement (about 43 versus 27 percent for placebo) at a dose of 150 mg/day administered subcutaneously. At 24 weeks, there was slowing of radiographic progression as well.

Significantly fewer new erosions were noted in the actively treated subjects (1.4 versus 2.6 for placebo, $p = 0.0005$). Analysis at 24 and 48 weeks (utilizing the Genant modification of the Sharp scoring method) revealed a retardation of radiographic progression as assessed by both erosions and joint space narrowing [78, 79]. A 24-week, double-blind randomized controlled trial of 419 patients involved multiple dosing regimens to assess the benefit of combining daily, subcutaneous anakinra with methotrexate in patients with active disease despite treatment with methotrexate. ACR 20, 50, and 70 percent responses were achieved in 42, 24, and 10 percent of patients who received combination therapy (at a dose of 1.0 mg/kg of anakinra), respectively [80].

How about side effects?

Transient injection site reactions were the most frequent adverse effects reported, resulting in a five percent withdrawal rate, though serious infections can occur. A higher serious infection rate has been observed in patients receiving the combination of etanercept and anakinra, leading to an FDA warning about combining these two agents [81]. Although the combination of anakinra and anti-TNF-alpha therapies should be avoided, it appears that anakinra can be added with relative safety to other DMARD therapies, including methotrexate, hydroxychloroquine, sulfasalazine, leflunomide, or azathioprine. Anakinra is generally used after failure of one to three anti-TNF agents. It is modestly effective in improving signs and symptoms as well as inhibiting radiographic progression in rheumatoid arthritis.

Two new members of the arsenal against rheumatoid arthritis are rituximab, which inhibits B cells, and abatacept, which inhibits T cell costimulation. See the chapter on rheumatoid arthritis for further discussion of these medications.

Staphylococcal Protein A Column

The staphylococcal protein A column is a silica column on which staphylococcal protein A is absorbed. The patient's blood is run through the column at a blood bank facility with experience in pheresis technique [82]. This method of immunoabsorption ameliorates the signs and symptoms of rheumatoid arthritis [83]. An important caveat is that patients on angiotensin converting enzyme inhibitors must not use this method of treatment, as their blood pressure will drop precipitously.

The DMARDS and biological agents require safety monitoring (Table 1).

Table 1. Monitoring Selected DMARD and Biological Therapy for Toxicity

DMARD/Biological	Monitor for	At Baseline	During Therapy
Sulfasalazine	Bone marrow suppression	CBC; ALT; G6PD level	CBC every two-four weeks for the first three mo, then every three mo
Hydroxychloroquine	Macular damage	Funduscopy and Amsler grid for loss of red perception	Annual ophth. exam
Methotrexate	Bone marrow suppression; liver fibrosis; pneumonitis	CBC; ALT and AST; albumin(1); BUN and creatinine; CXR; hepatitis B and C serologies	CBC; ALT and AST; serum albumin every eight weeks
Leflunomide	Hepatotoxicity Thrombocytopenia	ALT and AST; CBC	ALT and AST; CBC every eight weeks
Infliximab Etanercept Adalimumab	Infections, including TB	CBC; PPD, ?CXR	CBC every four months. Vigilance for infection
Anakinra	Neutropenia	Neutrophil count	Neutrophil counts every mo for the first three mo, then every three mo for one year

Reference: St. Clair EW: Disease-modifying antirheumatic drugs. In Klippel JH, Crofford LJ, Stone JH, Weyand CM (eds): Primer on the Rheumatic Diseases, 12th ed. Atlanta, Arthritis Foundation, 2001, pp 599-606.

Abbreviations: CBC, complete blood count; ALT, alanine aminotransferase; AST, aspartate aminotransferase; G6PD, glucose 6-phosphate dehydrogenase; PPD, purified protein derivative; CXR, chest X-ray

Footnotes: 1) Low serum albumin allows increased free methotrexate levels.

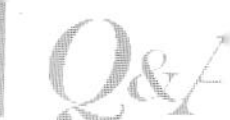

CALCITONIN – A MEDICATION WITH MULTIPLE PURPOSES

What is calcitonin?

Calcitonin is a 32-amino acid polypeptide that is secreted by the parafollicular cells of the thyroid gland in mammals[84]. Calcitonin plays a crucial role in the regulation of calcium and phosphate. In humans, serum calcium levels control the secretion of calcitonin. Calcitonin is commercially available as the human and salmon hormones, which differ slightly in their amino acid sequences. However, their pharmacological activity is the same. The salmon preparation is preferred because its duration of action is longer, and salmon calcitonin is approximately fifty times more potent than the human preparation. Furthermore, human calcitonin forms a thick gel that theoretically might limit its therapeutic usefulness.

How does calcitonin work?

Calcitonin acts primarily on bone, but it also affects the kidneys and gastrointestinal tract to lower serum calcium. Serum calcium levels directly control calcitonin secretion; as serum calcium levels increase, so does calcitonin. Calcitonin then binds to calcitonin receptors on osteoclasts, causing a marked decrease in their activity and number. This effect is transient after a single dose, but becomes prolonged with continued therapy. Calcitonin exerts its inhibitory effect on osteoclasts by increasing levels of intracellular cyclic adenosine monophosphate (cAMP). The cAMP, in turn, inhibits the release of intracellular calcium through unclear mechanisms[85]. In addition, when osteoclasts are exposed to calcitonin, they retract and loosen from the bone surface. Calcitonin may also promote bone accretion by increasing osteoblastic activity; however, the exact relationship between calcitonin and osteoblasts has not been established. Renal function is also altered by calcitonin. Renal excretion of filtered calcium, phosphate, sodium, magnesium, chloride, and potassium is increased by decreasing tubular resorption of these ions[84]. Some patients, however, may actually experience a decrease in urinary calcium because the decreased bone resorption overrides the increased renal excretion. Calcitonin also significantly affects the gastrointestinal tract by decreasing gastric acidity and decreasing the secretion of digestive peptides from the pancreas[86]. It is unclear how these effects relate to serum calcium levels.

How is calcitonin administered and what is the correct dosage?

Calcitonin salmon can be administered either intravenously, intramuscularly, subcutaneously, or nasally. There is no oral form of the drug; since it is a polypeptide, gastric enzymes easily digest it. When calcitonin salmon is administered nasally, the patient should be instructed to alternate nostrils daily. Patients appreciate the ease of administration of the nasal spray. The intranasal dose is one spray daily, which is equivalent to 200 Iµ of calcitonin per day. The parenteral dose is between 50 and 100 Iµ daily.

How well is calcitonin salmon absorbed?

When calcitonin salmon is administered parenterally, it is absorbed directly into the circulation. Following intravenous administration, the onset of action is immediate. It takes approximately 15 minutes for calcitonin salmon to start working when given intramuscularly or subcutaneously[84]. It has been shown that calcitonin salmon is absorbed rapidly by the nasal mucosa when it is given as a nasal spray. Peak plasma concentrations occur approximately 35 minutes after nasal dosing. The intranasal dose is about 40% as potent as a parenteral dose[86].

How is calcitonin salmon metabolized?

The metabolism of calcitonin salmon has not been studied extensively, but it is believed that the drug is rapidly metabolized by conversion to smaller, inactive peptides. A very small amount of unchanged calcitonin (0.1%) is excreted in the urine.

What are the main indications for calcitonin?

Both salmon and human calcitonin is used in the management of moderate to severe Paget's disease of the bone (osteitis deformans) and in osteoporosis. By interfering with osteoclasts, calcitonin causes a decreased rate of bone resorption. In Paget's disease of the bone, there is a subsequent fall in urine markers of bone resorption, as well as serum alkaline phosphatase. Also, patients who are treated with calcitonin usually experience less bone pain. Calcitonin has an analgesic effect on osteoporotic compression fractures as well.

In Paget's disease of the bone, there can be improved auditory nerve and neurologic function, regression of bone lesions radiographically, and correction of the high cardiac output with calcitonin treatment. However, while

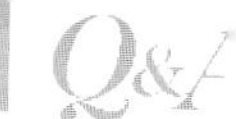

decreased bone pain is frequently seen with therapy, the other benefits are less predictable [87]. Calcitonin salmon nasal spray is useful in postmenopausal osteoporosis. The nasal spray was approved for the treatment of postmenopausal osteoporosis by the FDA in 1995. However, the data on the drug's efficacy is still somewhat controversial. Calcitonin nasal spray increases bone mineral density, particularly in the spine, as measured by dual energy X-ray absorptiometry (DEXA). A randomized, double-blinded study in 1997 showed a 6.8% increase in bone mineral density (BMD) after six months and an 11% increase after 12 months of therapy. In contrast, there was a 3.3% and a 5% decrease in BMD in the placebo group at six and 12 months, respectively. These were mean values in BMD as measured in the lumbar spine, cervical spine, ward's triangle, and trochanteric area of the hip. All patients in this study received one gram of daily calcium supplementation [88].

Although, calcitonin salmon does increase BMD, it has not yet been shown unequivocally to decrease the fracture rate, although, one study did suggest this effect [89]. Obviously, a decrease in fractures is the ultimate goal of therapy. Some studies demonstrate that the effect of salmon calcitonin seems to wane after 12 months of therapy. Finally, for unclear reasons, calcitonin does not seem to work well in early post-menopausal patients, so it is reserved for patients that are five or more years postmenopausal.

Calcitonin salmon can also be used in the early treatment of hypercalcemic emergencies, along with other appropriate agents. Either the injectable or nasal preparation can be used, but the parenteral form is somewhat more effective. It has been shown to decrease serum calcium levels in hypercalcemic patients with carcinoma, multiple myeloma, or primary hyperparathyroidism. However, patients with the latter tend to have a lesser response.

What are other less common indications for calcitonin salmon?

Glucocorticoid-induced osteoporosis is a vexing problem. The effects of calcitonin salmon have been studied in patients treated with glucocorticoids because of glucocorticoid-induced bone resorption. Several studies indicate that calcitonin salmon maintains or produces a small increase in bone density in these patients. One trial demonstrated beneficial effects of calcitonin salmon in patients with adhesive capsulitis of the shoulder. This study suggested that a combination of calcitonin salmon and physical therapy was significantly better in relieving pain than physical therapy alone [90]. Calcitonin salmon has also provided sustained pain relief in some patients with reflex sympathetic dystrophy (RSD). Treatment of RSD with calcitonin salmon is usually done via parenteral administration [91, 92].

How does calcitonin exert its analgesic effect?

This seems to be a centrally mediated mechanism. Several randomized, placebo-controlled trials demonstrate that salmon calcitonin has an analgesic effect on patients with acute vertebral compression fractures [93]. Pain relief usually occurs in the first two weeks of therapy and can continue for as long as four months with maintenance therapy.

What about calcitonin's side effects?

Calcitonin salmon is safe and generally well tolerated. When given parenterally, side effects can include mild nausea, flushing, and local irritation at the injection site. Calcitonin salmon nasal spray is generally well tolerated too, with occasional rhinitis, nasal dryness and crusts as potential side effects [94, 95].

Anabolic Bone Agents for Severe, Recalcitrant Osteoporosis

An interesting development in the treatment of osteoporosis is the use of recombinant human parathyroid hormone. A feature of hyperparathyroidism is osteoporosis, but cyclical use of the 1-34 amino acid fragment, from the amino terminal, of recombinant parathormone (rhPTH 1-34), or the entire 84 amino acid molecule, has an *anabolic* effect on bone [96]. RhPTH 1-34 administration reverses osteoporotic bone defects without compromising cortical bone strength [97]. A meta-analysis of randomized trials reports that this therapy increased spine bone density, decreased vertebral fractures, and decreased nonvertebral fractures [98]. Teriparatide should be used only for women and men at high risk of fracture. High-risk individuals include those who have failed prior treatment, those who had a previous osteoporotic fracture, or those who have multiple risk factors for fracture. Teriparatide is administered subcutaneously, 20 mcg once daily, into the thigh or abdominal wall. Initial administration should occur where the patient can sit or lie down in case of orthostatic hypotension. Headache, nausea and flushing might occur with the initiation of the injections, but abate after a few weeks. It is important to monitor serum calcium levels. Use of teriparatide for more than two years is not recommended, as its safety and efficacy have not been evaluated beyond this time. A theoretical concern is osteosarcoma, which occurs in rats and is

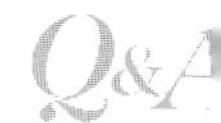

dose and duration dependent. Bone mineral density is lost after teriparatide treatment is stopped. However, giving a bisphosphonate after teriparatide treatment is stopped seems to be beneficial in maintaining the gain[99].

It is to be emphasized not to co-administer a bisphosphonate with teriparatide, as bisphosphonates interfere with the anabolic bone effects of teriparatide[100]. Osteonecrosis of the mandible from bisphosphonates is a concern. Most patients received intravenous bisphosphonates for malignancy, and dental hygiene seems to be an important predisposing factor.
The study of sodium flouride as an anabolic agent for bone has had a long, disappointing history. The quality of bone from treatment with sodium fluoride has been problematic, with weak bone and no improvement in fracture rates. However, low dose, slow-release fluorides, or use of sodium monofluorophosphate (MFP), may yet prove beneficial[101,102].

GLUCOCORTICOIDS

Who introduced the use of glucocorticoids to medicine?

The glucocorticoids are virtually "miracle drugs," albeit their use is a double-edged sword. After Drs. Philip S. Hench and Edward C. Kendall were awarded the Nobel Prize in 1950 for the isolation and first clinical use of cortisone at the Mayo Clinic, the dire side effects of its long-term, unbridled use became all too apparent to the medical community.

What can the glucocorticoids do <u>for</u> our patients?

The glucocorticoids are potent antiinflammatory agents. Employed judiciously, their use in rheumatology has facilitated control of many of the noninfectious inflammatory diseases. However, they should be used for the shortest duration and at the lowest dose to achieve disease control, and then tapered off.
For rheumatologic emergencies, for example imminently life-threatening or sight-threatening disease such as acute proliferative glomerulonephritis in systemic lupus erythematosus, life-threatening rheumatoid vasculitis, or giant cell arteritis with symptoms of impending loss of vision (e.g. blurred vision), methylprednisolone can be used at the very high dose of 1000 mg intravenously daily for three consecutive days, so called pulse-therapy, followed by oral prednisone or prednisolone at one mg kg/day. Generally, the dose of

prednisone or prednisolone for vital organ inflammation that is not imminently life or function threatening is 1 mg/kg per day, and tapered as soon as disease control permits. A discrete end-point must be identified, for instance one month for giant cell arteritis or six months for the systemic necrotizing vasculitides, and then the glucocorticoid tapered off.

Rheumatoid arthritis might be an exception, where low dose glucocorticoid therapy, 7.5 mg or less of prednisone or prednisolone each morning, might be continued long term in combination with other therapy. Glucocorticoids are the mainstays of treatment for polymyalgia rheumatica and giant cell arteritis. See the respective sections for details.

What are the anti-inflammatory mechanisms of action of the glucocorticoids?

Inflammatory stress stimulates production of proinflammatory cytokines, such as tumor necrosis factor-alpha, interleukin-1 and interleukin-6. These cytokines in turn stimulate the production of hydrocortisone to limit inflammation and tissue damage in a feedback loop. The glucocorticoids exert their antiinflammatory actions by diverse mechanisms. Some of these mechanisms are suppression of proinflammatory cytokine production, inhibition of T-lymphocyte and macrophage function, inhibition of migration of neutrophils and monocytes to areas of inflammation, and suppression of prostaglandin E2 and leukotriene formation. Interestingly, glucocorticoids have little effect on mature, antibody forming B cells.

What is nuclear factor-kappa B and what is the role of glucocorticoids in suppressing this factor?

Nuclear factor-kappa B, (NF-kB) is a key transcription factor that plays a pivotal role in the activation of many genes important in the production of some mediators of inflammation. TNF-alpha, and IL-6 are examples of such mediators. NF-kB is found in the cytoplasm of cells in an inactive form coupled to an inhibitory protein called IkappaBeta. Extracellular stimuli cause phosphorylation of IkappaB, permitting NF-kB to migrate to the cell nucleus and bind its target genes to initiate transcription. Glucocorticoids induce the synthesis of a protein that inactivates nuclear factor-kappa B.

What can the glucocorticoids do to our patients, and how can we reduce the risk?

Glucocorticoid toxicities are legion and must be monitored. HPA axis suppression, osteoporosis with vertebral compression fractures, infections, diabetes mellitus, hypertension, cataracts, and glaucoma are among the feared consequences of chronic, therapeutic doses of a glucocorticoid. Several tapering regimens have been advocated. One such tapering program is as follows: When the dose of prednisone or prednisolone is more than 40 mg/day, or equivalent of another glucocorticoid (Table 2), decrease the dose by 5 to 10 mg (or equivalent) every one to two weeks. Then, at a dose of prednisone or prednisolone between 40 and 20 mg/day, or equivalent, taper by 5 mg or equivalent every one to two weeks. At a dose of prednisone or prednisolone of less than 20 mg/day (or equivalent), taper by 1 to 2.5 mg/day (or equivalent) every two to three weeks. It is important to monitor for a disease flare, and go to the next higher dose if indicated. Patients with rheumatoid arthritis are particularly sensitive to steroid tapering, and a tapering schedule as slow as one mg a month, or even 1/2 mg a month or every six weeks, might have to be used.

There are other strategies to lessen the toxicity of glucocorticoid therapy. For severe disease resistant to glucocorticoids, use a steroid-sparing medication concomitantly, e.g., methotrexate or azathioprine for an idiopathic inflammatory myositis, or cyclophosphamide for a systemic necrotizing vasculitis or proliferative glomerulonephritis in systemic lupus erythematosus. In the inflammatory rheumatic diseases, if necessary and if possible, eventual alternate day glucocorticoid treatment should be the aim to maintain disease control because it is attended by less toxicity. To try to avoid glucocorticoid-induced osteoporosis, it is very important to use concomitant calcium (1,500 mg daily of elemental calcium in two divided doses for better absorption) and vitamin D (800 IU daily), as well as a bisphosphonate in some cases.

The use of a bisphosphonate in patients newly started on a glucocorticoid, prednisone or prednisolone 5 mg per day or higher, or equivalent, with an anticipated duration of therapy of three months or longer, is recommended by the American College of Rheumatology to prevent glucocorticoid-induced osteoporosis [103]. Alendronate (5 mg daily or 35 mg once a week) or risedronate (5 mg daily or 35 mg once a week) are effective in the prevention and treatment of glucocorticoid-induced bone loss and are approved by the Federal Drug Administration for this use. For patients already on chronic glucocorticoid therapy, a DEXA study should be performed annually, and a bisphosphonate started if the T score is less than –1 [103]. Risk factors for osteoporosis should be aggressively controlled, e.g., smoking and alcohol consumption. Consider a proton pump inhibitor for gastrointestinal protection, especially if an NSAID is being used concomitantly with a glucocorticoid.

It must be kept in mind that the HPA axis can be blunted for about a year after chronic glucocorticoid therapy is tapered, and a stress situation, such as pneumonia or major surgery, can precipitate acute adrenal insufficiency. Stress doses of hydrocortisone are given in such circumstances. One regimen is to give 100 mg of hydrocortisone intravenously every six hours for three days. If the patient is judged to be at low risk of adrenal insufficiency, e.g., having used ≤7.5 mg daily of prednisone or prednisolone for less than approximately three months, give 50 mg of hydrocortisone intravenously on the day of surgery, followed by 25 to 50 mg of hydrocortisone intravenously every eight hours for two or three days. If the patient has a minor febrile illness, doubling the dose of glucocorticoid for about three days will suffice, and the patient should be instructed to call his health care provider for further evaluation. Please note, a drop in blood pressure might signal the need for more glucocorticoid. Remember that the serum potassium is usually misleadingly normal in such situations because the zona glomerulosa is less suppressed by exogenous glucocorticoids, and aldosterone is relatively unaffected.

Table 2. Equivalent Doses of Various Glucocorticoids

Drug	Equivalent dose (mg)
Hydrocortisone (cortisol, the form produced by the adrenal glands)	20
Cortisone	25
Prednisone and prednisolone	5
Methylprednisolone	4
Triamcinolone	4
Dexamethasone	0.75
Betamethasone	0.6

When feasible, and in the absence of infection, soft tissue and intrarticular glucocorticoid injection therapy can be very effective in suppressing inflammation in a local site, and with less systemic toxicity[104]. We refer the reader to a textbook of rheumatology for more detail on soft tissue and joint injection therapy for the rheumatic diseases.

KEY POINTS

- Methotrexate is currently the disease modifying antirheumatic drug (DMARD) of choice for rheumatoid arthritis as well as several other rheumatic diseases.
- It is often used in combination with other antirheumatic agents for recalcitrant disease.
- Hydroxychloroquine is an essential adjunct for systemic lupus erythematosus, decreasing disease flares.
- To minimize the risk of hydroxychloroquine retinopathy, do not exceed a dose of 6.5 mg/kg/day, ideal body weight.
- Sulfasalazine is an effective DMARD for rheumatoid arthritis and the spondyloarthritides.
- Leflunomide, a pyrimidine inhibitor, is indicated for moderate to severe, active rheumatoid arthritis.
- It is now strongly recommended to initiate aggressive, combination DMARD therapy after six weeks, but before 12 weeks, of active, refractory rheumatoid arthritis.
- The biologic antirheumatic agents, the tumor necrosis factor-alpha blockers etanercept, infliximab and adalimumab, and the interleukin-1 blocker anakinra, have opened an exciting new era in the treatment of the rheumatic diseases.
- Calcitonin can help ameliorate the bone pain of an osteoporotic compression fracture.
- Teriparatide, a parathormone analogue, is a novel anabolic agent for selected patients with severe osteoporosis.

CHAPTER 31

THE CLINICAL LABORATORY IN RHEUMATOLOGY

Mitchel J Seleznick

SYNOVIAL FLUID ANALYSIS

What essential tests should be performed on synovial fluid after arthrocentesis?

It is essential to note volume and clarity, and to perform a Gram stain and culture, a white cell count and differential as well as a polarized light examination for crystals. The gross appearance of synovial fluid can give an approximation of the white cell count. Clear joint fluid indicates a low leukocyte count, such as in osteoarthritis. Translucent joint fluid, through which one can see, is consistent with mildly inflammatory arthritis, such as in systemic lupus erythematosus. Opalescent or opaque synovial fluid is indicative of intense inflammation and a very high leukocyte count, such as one sees in septic arthritis.

Some time-honored tests are no longer considered of use. These tests include glucose, protein, lactate, synovial fluid viscosity, mucin clot, and immunologic tests, such as synovial fluid rheumatoid factor, antinuclear antibody test or complement levels.

What diagnoses can be made based on synovial fluid analysis?

A definitive diagnosis of infection and crystal deposition arthritis disease can be made by synovial fluid analysis[1]. An exception is Neisseria gonorrhoeae, which usually cannot be cultured reliably. Synovial fluid analysis is necessary to make a definitive diagnosis of crystal deposition arthritis[2]. Monosodium urate crystals are needle shaped and strongly (shine brightly under polarized light) negatively birefringent, appearing yellow when parallel to the axis of slow vibration of a first order red compensator, and blue when perpendicular. Conversely, calcium pyrophosphate dihydrate (CPPD) crystals are rhomboid-shaped and weakly positively birefringent, appearing blue when parallel to the compensator and yellow when perpendicular[3]. The presence of these crystals within synovial fluid polymorphonuclear leukocytes is pathognomonic of an attack of gouty arthritis (Figure 1) or CPPD crystal deposition disease (pseudogout) respectively. It should be pointed out that the CPPD crystals are easy to miss and have to be looked for carefully.

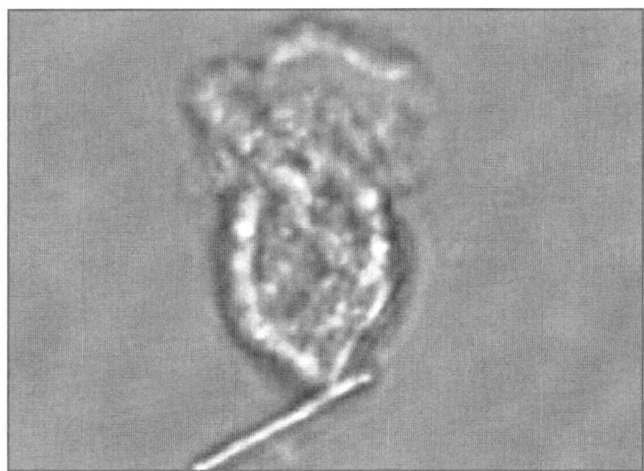

Figure 1. *Study of synovial fluid in gout: Contact between a urate crystal and a polymorphonuclear leucocyte.*

DeAngelis R, Grassi WW, Cervini C. University of Ancona, Italy

What crystals other than urate and pyrophosphate cause arthritis and may be seen in synovial fluid?

A variety of other crystals may be seen in synovial fluid. *Basic calcium phosphate crystals*, principally hydroxyapatite, are found commonly in patients with connective tissue diseases, renal disease, osteoarthritis, and in the Milwaukee Shoulder-Knee syndrome. These crystals are too minuscule to be identified by light microscopy, although they may be seen as rounded, coin-like aggregates if they are clumped together.

Cholesterol crystals may be seen in any chronic inflammatory effusion, and are mostly seen in rheumatoid arthritis. Lipid crystals may be seen in association with joint trauma and have a Maltese cross appearance. *Calcium oxalate crystals* have a characteristic bipyramidal appearance and are commonly found in patients with renal disease and in primary hyperoxaluria, especially in patients who supplement their diet with ascorbic acid. *Steroid crystals* exhibit both positive and negative birefringence and can be seen in synovial fluid following intraarticular steroid injection.

How is the synovial fluid cell count interpreted?

The cell count is a measure of inflammation and is very helpful in the classification of joint fluid. Cell counts less than 2,000 WBC/hpf are considered non-inflammatory. Cell counts greater than 100,000 are to be considered septic until proven otherwise. Septic synovial fluids usually have greater than 50,000 white blood cells. There is considerable overlap between infectious and inflammatory cell counts. The differential count is also useful in that in septic arthritis, greater than 95% of cells are polymorphonuclear leukocytes, while in RA, less than 90% of cells are polymorphonuclear leukocytes. Noninflammatory joint fluids will have <50% polymorphonuclear leukocytes[3]. It is important to note that synovial fluid has to be examined shortly after being aspirated from the joint. The white cell count may spuriously decrease within hours, obscuring an inflammatory process. Calcium pyrophosphate dihydrate crystals change shape and their birefringence characteristics within 24 hours of arthrocentesis. Monosodium urate crystals change only slightly with time. Thus, prompt examination of synovial fluid is essential to avoid losing characteristic findings.

RHEUMATOID FACTOR

What is rheumatoid factor, and how is it measured?

Rheumatoid factor (RF) is an antibody against an antibody directed against the Fc portion of one's own IgG. Although any class of immunoglobulin may have this property, clinical laboratories commonly report only IgM rheumatoid factors. RF has traditionally been measured by the latex fixation test in which latex particles are coated with IgG and agglutinate in the presence of RF. Clinical labs are now using an enzyme-linked immunosorbent assay, or ELISA, and nephelometry to try to improve reliability. A nephelometer quantifies the degree of turbidity or light reflected through a sample. In the case of rheumatoid factor, the turbidity is produced by an antigen-antibody interaction in serum.

What is the sensitivity and specificity of rheumatoid factor for rheumatoid arthritis?

The sensitivity has been estimated to be 0.75-0.9: rheumatoid factor is positive in 75-90% of patients with RA[4]. However, it is a non-specific test and can be present in many other chronic inflammatory conditions[5]. Examples of these conditions are systemic lupus erythematosus, Sjögren syndrome, mixed cryoglobulinemia, sarcoidosis, subacute bacterial endocarditis, chronic liver disease, tuberculosis, Lyme disease, acquired immunodeficiency disease, and parasitic diseases, some of which cause arthritis. In addition, the rate of false positivity increases with age [6-8].

What is the clinical utility of the new anti-cyclic citrullinated peptides (CCP) assay?

The anti-CCP assay is a test that is more specific than rheumatoid factor for rheumatoid arthritis, 90.4% vs 80.3%. It is less sensitive, though, 66% vs about 72%. If both anti-CCP and rheumatoid factor assays are used, testing sensitivity for RA increases to 81.4%, as 34% of rheumatoid factor negative rheumatoid arthritis patients were positive for anti-CCP antibodies. Furthermore, anti-CCP antibodies correlate with a more destructive, erosive course of RA. This test is becoming more widely available [9].

OTHER AUTO-ANTIBODIES

How are antinuclear antibodies (ANAs) used in the evaluation of a patient with possible connective tissue disease?

As for the rheumatoid factor, proper interpretation of ANA results depends on the *pre-test probability* of disease. The normal population has a 2-5% false positive rate; therefore, ANA tests should not be used for screening asymptomatic people. In a patient with multisystem illness or features of connective tissue disease, a *negative* ANA will tend to *rule* out the diagnosis of SLE. In a patient with Raynaud's phenomenon, a positive ANA is predictive of a systemic rheumatic disease [10]. Thus, a positive ANA is consistent with, but not specific for SLE. Patients with Sjogren's syndrome, mixed connective tissue disease (MCTD), and scleroderma have high frequencies of positive ANAs. On the other hand, antibodies against double-stranded, or native, DNA and Smith antigens are very specific for SLE [11]. Other applications of autoantibodies include high-titer anti-RNP, which is highly sensitive for MCTD [11], and anti-Ro (SS-A) and anti-La (SS-B) antibodies, seen in primary Sjögren's syndrome (70% and 50% respectively) and in SLE (30% and 15% respectively) [12]. Other Anti-Ro-associated syndromes include subacute cutaneous lupus and the neonatal lupus syndrome [12, 13], which includes complete heart block.

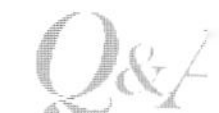

What other auto-antibodies are seen in association with rheumatic disease?

Other auto-antibody associations include anti-centromere antibodies in limited scleroderma (CREST syndrome) (50% sensitive for limited scleroderma; 2-15% in systemic sclerosis), anti-topoisomerase I antibodies (formerly anti-Scl-70 antibodies) in systemic sclerosis (40% sensitivity and 85% specific for systemic sclerosis; seen in about 15% of patients with limited scleroderma), and the anti-transfer RNA synthetases, most often anti-histidyl-tRNA synthetase (Jo-1) antibodies, in polymyositis or dermatomyositis [14-16]. Patients with poly or dermatomyositis and anti-Jo-1 antibodies are likely to have the constellation of interstitial pulmonary fibrosis, symmetric nonerosive arthritis, fever, "mechanic's hands" (cracked skin on the sides of the fingers), and Raynaud's phenomenon. This constellation is known as the anti-synthetase syndrome [16].

The anti-neutrophilic cytoplasmic antibodies, ANCAs, have been associated with a number of disorders, most notably Wegener's granulomatosis and pauci-immune glomerulonephritis. cANCA, for cytoplasmic antineutrophil cytoplasmic antibody, exhibits cytoplasmic staining and may be positive in greater that 90% of patients with active, diffuse Wegener's syndrome [17]. The antigen to which cANCA forms is a serine protease, proteinase3. pANCA, for peri-nuclear antineutrophil cytoplasmic antibody, exhibits perinuclear staining and is seen in pauci-immune glomerulonephritis and in other necrotizing vasculitides, including microscopic polyangiitis and Churg-Strauss syndrome [18]. The antigen to which pANCA forms in these patients is myeloperoxidase. Drug-induced, pANCA-positive vasculitis occurs most often from propylthiouracil or hydralazine [19].

What are the clinical correlates of anti-phospholipid antibodies?

The lupus anticoagulant, anticardiolipin antibodies, and antibodies causing a chronic false positive VDRL, are all antiphospholipid antibodies. The first two may be associated with venous and arterial thromboses, recurrent spontaneous abortion and thrombocytopenia [20] *the anti-phospholipid syndrome*. These antibodies may act at phospholipid epitopes in the coagulation cascade, including prothrombin and *beta2-glycoprotein I*, causing a hypercoagulable or thrombophilic state [21]. Antiphospholipid antibodies may be seen in association with SLE and other autoimmune syndromes, malignancies, infections, or in the absence of any other disease (the primary antiphospholipid syndrome). The lupus anticoagulant typically causes an elevated aPTT that does not correct with the addition of normal plasma. If necessary, confirmation of a lupus anticoagulant is by the Russell viper venom test or platelet neutralization test[22]. Anticardiolipin antibodies are detected by ELISA, the enzyme-linked immunosorbent assay.

COMPLEMENT

Are complement studies useful in following lupus patients?

A drop in complement components or a rise in complement activation products has been observed prior to disease flares in patients with lupus nephritis. Complement activation components include C3a and SC5b-9, and a rise in these components presages a flare in lupus nephritis earlier than a drop in C4, C3 or CH50. Consequently, they are useful in monitoring disease activity in individual lupus patients[23]. Complement components that are commonly measured are C3, C4, and CH50. CH50 is the level of total complement necessary to lyse 50% of sheep red blood cells sensitized with rabbit antibody. All nine components of the complement cascade are required for a normal CH50 level. It is a useful screening tool for detecting a homozygous deficiency of a component (C1 through C8) because complete deficiency of a given complement component will render CH50 undetectable. CH50 should be assayed when an appropriate patient is first seen because it screens for a component deficiency as well as for complement activation. In fact, homozygous deficiencies of C4 and C2 are associated with the development of an SLE-like syndrome[24].

ERYTHROCYTE SEDIMENTATION RATE (ESR)

How is the ESR best utilized in the diagnosis and management of rheumatic diseases?

The ESR by Westergren method, an *indirect* measure of acute phase reactants, mostly fibrinogen, is a non-specific test that is especially useful in the diagnosis and management of polymyalgia rheumatica (PMR), giant cell arteritis (GCA), paraproteinemias, and osteomyelitis[25]. Although PMR and GCA are characteristically associated with an elevated ESR, the ESR may be within the normal range in up to 20% of patients [26]. The ESR has been commonly used as a marker for disease activity in rheumatoid arthritis in both clinical trials and clinical practice [27].

C-REACTIVE PROTEIN

What is the value of this acute phase reactant?

The C-reactive protein (CRP), so called for its reactivity with the C polysaccharide of the pneumococcus, is a *direct* acute phase reactant. The CRP rises mainly in response to inflammatory cytokines such as interleukin 6. The temporal relationship between a rise and fall in CRP and onset or remission of an inflammatory condition is closer than that of the ESR. CRP levels begin rising a few hours after tissue injury, and peak in 24 to 72 hours. Likewise, levels return promptly to normal with resolution of inflammation. Furthermore, the degree of elevation correlates with the degree of tissue damage, and can reach levels as high as one thousand times normal. Because of its greater sensitivity and responsiveness to disease control, some authorities suggest replacing the ESR with CRP in testing for inflammatory states. For example, some studies have shown that CRP is a better test for active polymyalgia rheumatica and giant cell arteritis than is the ESR [28]. As these two tests are complementary, though, many authorities now advocate using both in the diagnosis of polymyalgia rheumatica and giant cell arteritis. A relative downside is the greater time and cost of doing a quantitative CRP assay. Obesity causes a mild elevated in CRP, approximately by 0.3mg/dl, because adipose tissue contains interleukin 6 [29]. In another application, a high sensitivity C-RP for detecting risk of coronary artery inflammation is in use. Its usefulness in this regard is still being defined [30].

PROTEIN CRYOGLOBULINS

What disease processes are associated with the presence of cryoglobulinemia?

Cryoglobulins are immunoglobulins that precipitate upon incubation in vitro at 0-4°C for about 72 hours. Type I cryoglobulins are monoclonal, usually IgM, and occur in individuals with lymphoma or Waldenstrom's macroglobulinemia. Type

II cryoglobulins consist of monoclonal IgM rheumatoid factor bound to IgG [31]. Type III cryoglobulins, the most common, consist of polyclonal IgM rheumatoid factor bound to IgG. Type II and III cryoglobulins in the serum act as circulating immune complexes and present with the signs of cutaneous or systemic vasculitis, cryoglobulinemic vasculitis. Glomerulonephritis occurs in about half of these patients with mixed cryoglobulinemia. What was considered "essential" mixed cryoglobulinemia, or the Meltzer-Franklin syndrome, in the past, is now known to be caused by hepatitis C in most cases, and treatment of hepatitis C can ameliorate the manifestations of mixed cryoglobulinemia. Mixed cryoglobulins may also be found in other chronic infections, SLE and RA [32].

Reliability of the cryoglobulin assay depends strictly on proper specimen collection and handling. The specimen must be collected in a warm syringe, allowed to clot, and then the serum is separated at 37°C by centrifuge. The serum is then incubated at 0-4°C for about 72 hours, and the cryoprecipitate noted on the bottom of the test tube. The precipitate can be assayed for the type of cryoglobulin. Rheumatoid factor is positive in the serum of patients with mixed cryoglobulinemia, and hypocomplementemia, especially a low C4. The low C4 is easier to ascertain than cryoglobulins, and if clinically consistent with mixed cryoglobulinemia, supports the diagnosis.

IMMUNE COMPLEX ASSAYS

How are circulating immune complexes measured?

Several different assays are available to measure circulating immune complexes, including C1Q binding, conglutinin binding in solid phase, polyethylene glycol precipitation, and the Raji cell assay. Although useful in research, these assays are of doubtful clinical utility due to poor sensitivity, specificity, and intercorrelation between methods.

HUMAN LEUKOCYTE ANTIGENS

When should HLA-B27 status be investigated?

HLA-B27 is a class I molecule of the Major Histocompatibility Complex (MHC) that binds antigenic peptides to be *presented to CD8+ T cells*. The diagnosis of HLA-B27-associated arthropathies, principally ankylosing spondylitis and reactive arthritis, can usually be made on clinical and radiological grounds. However, in the patient with chronic back pain and stiffness, and equivocal sacroiliac X-ray changes, a positive HLA B27 supports a diagnosis of these spondyloarthritides [33]. HLA-B27 may also be useful in the evaluation of patients with uveitis or aortic regurgitation, known to be associated with the spondyloarthritides.

What other rheumatic diseases are associated with HLA loci?

Most rheumatic disease associations are with MHC Class II gene products at the HLA-DR, DQ, and DP loci. The HLA class II molecules *present antigenic peptides to CD4+ T cells*. Approximately 70% of Caucasoids with rheumatoid arthritis (RA) are positive for HLA-DR4, which may be a marker for more severe disease, and increases the relative risk of RA six fold [34]. The frequency of HLA-DR4 in normal Caucasoid in the United States is 25%. Polymyalgia rheumatica is also associated with HLA-DR4 [35]. Forty to fifty percent of patients with systemic lupus erythematosus are positive for HLA-DR2 or DR3, the presence of which increases the relative risk of lupus three fold. HLA-DR3 is also associated with Sjögren's syndrome and increases the relative risk five fold. HLA-B51 is associated with Behçet's syndrome in Japanese and Eastern Mediterranean patients, but not in North American populations [36]. In the spondyloarthritides, HLA assays are more of scientific rather than clinical relevance.

METABOLIC BONE DISEASE

What is the role of biochemical markers of bone turnover in assessing patients with osteoporosis or Paget's disease of the bone?

The clinical use of biochemical markers is controversial. Bone mineral density scanning by DEXA (dual X-ray absorptiometry) is currently the preferred method of monitoring patients with osteoporosis, but meaningful comparisons with prior studies may not be possible for up to two years. Biochemical markers will reflect response to therapy after several weeks. Serum levels of bone specific alkaline phosphatase, osteocalcin, and type I collagen propeptides are markers of bone formation. Urinary products of collagen degradation, such as pyridinoline cross-links of collagen, cross-linked N- and C- telopeptides, and hydroxyproline are markers of bone resorption [37].

KEY POINTS

- Laboratory tests in rheumatology are not sufficiently sensitive or specific to allow a definitive diagnosis in the vast majority of diseases.
- In systemic lupus erythematosus, the antinuclear antibody test is very sensitive, up to 98%, so a negative test makes the diagnosis highly unlikely. A positive anti-Smith, and somewhat less so an anti-n DNA antibody test, are very specific tests for systemic lupus erythematosus, so make the diagnosis highly probably if positive.
- Wegener's granulomatosus is usually associated with cANCA against proteinase 3, and microscopic polyangiitis and Churg Strauss syndrome is usually associated with pANCA against myeloperoxidase. As an exception to the rule, however, myeloperoxidase antibodies (pANCA) can be positive in Wegener's granulomatosis, and proteinase 3 antibodies (cANCA) can be positive in microscopic polyangiitis and the Churg-Strauss syndrome. The two tests are not positive in the same patient. Synovianalysis is a very important part of the diagnostic stratagem in rheumatology.
- Joint fluid analysis is particularly useful in identifying inflammation, with a fluid white count above 3000 per mm^3; infection, with a white count above 50,000 with 90% neutrophils and a positive Gram's stain and culture/sensitivity; and a crystal deposition arthropathy.
- In gouty arthritis, the monosodium urate crystals are needle-shaped and negatively birefringent. In calcium pyrophosphate crystal deposition disease ("pseudogout"), the crystals are rhomboid-shaped and weakly positively birefringent.
- A recent shift in the use of inflammatory markers has the quantitative C-reactive protein more sensitive and more in parallel with inflammatory activity than the time-honored erythrosedimentation rate. These tests complement each other in polymyalgia rheumatica and giant cell arteritis.
- A new test, the anti-cyclic citrullinated peptide (CCP) assay, is very helpful in its specificity and ruling in the diagnosis of rheumatoid arthritis. It also gauges prognosis in rheumatoid arthritis.

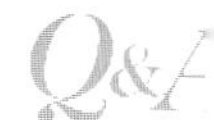

CHAPTER 32

FREQUENTLY ASKED QUESTIONS BY PATIENTS

Is arthritis curable yet?

There are about 100 different kinds of arthritis. The majority is not curable yet, but treatment is improving all the time, and we are able to control the different kinds of arthritis better now than even five years ago.

Is rheumatoid arthritis the "crippling kind" of arthritis and osteoarthritis the "non crippling" kind?

Both of these types of arthritis vary in severity and prognosis. Rheumatoid arthritis can be relatively mild and controllable, and some cases of osteoarthritis are severe and require surgery.

What about health food stores and natural herbs for arthritis?

There is no scientific proof that alternative methods help. However, ask your doctor about a given selection. As long as it is not injurious or does not interfere with the medications you are taking, it might be all right to try. Glucosamine and chondroitin sulfate may help some patients with osteoarthritis.

Is lupus fatal?

The prognosis of systemic lupus erythematosus has improved significantly in the past few decades. The 10-year survival rate is now about 90%. This improved outcome relates to earlier diagnosis and treatment, more effective control of lupus nephritis (kidney inflammation), and more effective use of antibiotics.

Are the anti-inflammatory drugs, the so-called "COX-2" inhibitors celecoxib and lumiracoxib, safer for the stomach than the first-generation nonsteroidal anti-inflammatory drugs (NSAIDs)? And is it more effective?

Celecoxib lumiracoxib are less injurious to the stomach, causing fewer ulcers and bleeding. They are more effective than the first generation antiinflammatory drugs. Currently, low dose celecoxib, 200 mg daily, is recommended for patients at high risk of gastrointestinal side effects, and at low risk for heart attack and stroke. This issue is being elucidated as of the writing of this book. Using an acid "pump inhibitor" is partially effective in protecting the stomach and duodenum for those who need an NSAID but are at risk of GI complications.

What happens if I stop my prednisone too fast?

Your blood pressure could drop dangerously low if you stop prednisone too fast. Make sure you follow your doctor's instructions carefully.

If I get too many injections into my joints, what can happen?

More than four injections into a weight-bearing joint, such as the knee, in one year is generally inadvisable. Too many joint injections may lead to further wearing out of the joint cartilage.

Clinoril works for my friend, but not for me. Why?

In general, there seems to be more of an art than a science to which nonsteroidal anti-inflammatory medication works best for a given individual. The reason for this observation is not clear. Thus, it is important to give an arthritis medication time to work, about two or three weeks, and if it is not effective, try another. Your doctor will guide you.

What should I watch out for with my arthritis medication?

All medications have side effects, some more than others. The nonsteroidal antiinflammatory drugs can cause various side effects, the most common of which are stomach irritation and sometimes ulcers that can bleed. If you experience heartburn or indigestion while on arthritis medication, tell your doctor. Likewise, it is imperative to tell your doctor at once if you notice black, sticky stool.

What causes tendinitis?

Tendinitis is generally caused by exertion or overuse. Treatment consists of rest, an antiinflammatory medication, and perhaps an injection of a cortisone-like medication near the tendon.

Is it dangerous to get pregnant if you have arthritis?

The answer to this question depends on several things. The clearest answer pertains to lupus. If a person with lupus has active disease that is not under control, especially if the kidneys are inflamed, pregnancy would be better postponed. Some patients with rheumatoid arthritis go into remission when they get pregnant; the arthritis comes back after delivery.

With all the tests that are available, shouldn't my doctor be able to diagnose my arthritis easily?

Not all the time. There are over 100 different reasons joints can hurt, and sometimes a doctor has to follow a patient for a while before a specific diagnosis can be made.

I've heard methotrexate is one of the best arthritis medications. Why doesn't my doctor use it for me?

Methotrexate is not effective for all kinds of arthritis. For instance, the most common arthritis, osteoarthritis, does not respond to this medication. Furthermore, methotrexate might be too dangerous for people with certain coexisting conditions. Your doctor can discuss your specific situation with you.

What is fibromyalgia?

Fibromyalgia is a common painful condition. Disturbed sleep is probably a contributing factor. Fibromyalgia is not crippling, but it can be quite painful. Treatment includes aerobic exercise and medication that promotes a certain stage of sleep.

What are the most common side effects of inhaled calcitonin?

The most frequent side effects are an occasional runny nose or nasal dryness.

Will calcitonin nasal spray give me sinusitis?

There is no increased rate of sinusitis in patients who use calcitonin.

Will the nasal spray affect my sense of smell?

No.

Does my body actually absorb the medication?

Yes. Your body absorbs the medication from the inner lining of your nose.

How does a nasal spray retard osteoporosis?

This medication retards the cells that break down your bones.

Why should I alternate nostrils daily when taking this medication?

This helps lessen the side effects.

Is this medication really derived from fish?

Yes. Calcitonin nasal spray is derived from salmon.

Does the medication smell like fish?

No. It has no odor.

What are the most common side effects of leflunomide?

The most common side effects include liver, bone marrow, or kidney problems. All of these are, however, rare. Some people also experience diarrhea from the drug, especially at higher doses.

Do I need to have my blood checked while I take this medication?

Yes. You should have your blood monitored approximately four weeks after beginning therapy and then every six to eight weeks thereafter.

Which of the aforementioned side effects is the most likely?

The most frequently seen side effect is liver toxicity.

Is the liver toxicity irreversible?

The liver toxicity most frequently resolves when the medication is discontinued. If the liver toxicity is mild, it usually resolves even if the medication is not stopped.

Is there an antidote for the toxicity?

No, although cholestyramine does hasten elimination of leflunomide from the body.

Can one get pregnant or father a child while taking this medication?

No, because leflunomide causes birth defects.

How long does the drug stay in my body once I stop taking it?

It can take several weeks, if not months, to fully eliminate leflunomide from your body once you stop taking the medication.

Is there a way to eliminate the drug from your body more quickly?

Yes. Your doctor can give you another medication, cholestyramine, that significantly increases the clearance of leflunomide from your body.

Does leflunomide work better than more conventional therapies for rheumatoid arthritis?

No, leflunomide compares favorably to methotrexate.

Can I take this medication with other drugs for rheumatoid arthritis?

Yes.

What are the most common side effects of etanercept?

The most frequent side effect is local irritation at the injection site. There is also a small increase in the rate of upper respiratory infections in patients taking etanercept.

Is there any liver toxicity associated with etanercept?

No. There have been no reports of liver, bone marrow, or kidney problems from this medication.

What kind of a medication is etanercept?

It is a genetically engineered tumor necrosis factor receptor.

What is a tumor necrosis factor receptor?

Tumor necrosis factor is a natural substance that everyone has in his or her body. It helps mediate inflammation. Etanercept is actually a soluble receptor for tumor necrosis factor. Thus, it acts as a "sponge" for tumor necrosis factor and thereby decreases inflammation.

Are there potential harmful effects of negating tumor necrosis factor?

Possibly. A patient taking etanercept may be at slightly increased risk of infection (especially upper respiratory infections). Also, as the name would imply, tumor necrosis factor may protect against tumors. Both of these concerns have been closely monitored. There is no clear indication that tumor necrosis factor inhibition increases the likelihood of life threatening infections or increased rates of cancer.

Does this medication come in the form of a pill?

No. It has to be administered by an injection just under the skin.

How often do I have to take the shot?

It is administered once or twice weekly.

Does etanercept work better than conventional therapies for rheumatoid arthritis?

Results so far are very encouraging. Etanercept works as well as methotrexate, and some studies suggest that it works better. Combination therapy with methotrexate is clearly the most effective regimen.

How long does it take the medication to work?

Most patients start to notice relief within two to four weeks of initiating therapy.

Will the benefit of etanercept "wear off" after months or years of use?

This has yet to be determined.

Will I become crippled or deformed by the arthritis?

If the arthritis destroys cartilage or bone, called erosive arthritis, it can cause deformities. The deformities from erosive rheumatoid arthritis can now be stopped or at least delayed. Furthermore, pain and swelling from inflammation can be treated and significantly controlled using many different anti-inflammatory medications. Sometimes, chronic arthritis may result in such pain and loss of function that joint replacement is indicated. Joint replacement can provide remarkable relief and restoration of function. Curiously, the degree of pain does not necessarily correlate with the degree of joint destruction or likelihood of deformity.

Is my disease genetic?

Many rheumatic diseases (e.g. lupus, rheumatoid arthritis) have genetic components. Some unusual rheumatic diseases, such as Familial Mediterranean Fever, have actually been traced to a specific gene mutation. However, the more common rheumatic diseases such as osteoarthritis, rheumatoid arthritis, and lupus are likely combinations of unidentified genetic and environmental factors. Clustering of these diseases within families does exist, and a family medical history is important in making a diagnosis in some cases.

What is the chance my children will get my arthritis?

Although, as noted above, there are genetic elements to many of the rheumatic disease, in general, transmission to offspring is not very common. The chance that a patient with rheumatoid arthritis or lupus will give birth to a child who will develop the same disease is very low, although somewhat higher than that of a parent without arthritis.

Can I have children?

Although patients with lupus were once told never to have children, this is no longer necessarily the case. However, a patient with uncontrolled lupus or other severe rheumatic disease should not become pregnant until their disease is well controlled or in remission. Some rheumatic diseases can flare during pregnancy, some may flare postpartum, and some can go into remission during pregnancy. Furthermore, many of the drugs we use to treat the rheumatic diseases can harm the fetus or cause fertility problems. Communication between the patient and their rheumatologist is a very important part of family planning.

Why can't anyone tell me exactly what my diagnosis is?

Many rheumatic diseases are defined by a set of clinical and laboratory data. Often, it takes more than one doctor visit or set of laboratory findings to allow a specific diagnosis. Sometimes, a patient's problems may not fit any specific disease definition, or may overlap between a number of different diagnoses. Furthermore, early disease can present with nonspecific signs and symptoms. In such cases, a rheumatologist may require time to see what develops over months or sometimes even years.

Will I need to take this medication for the rest of my life?

Most rheumatic diseases are chronic and do require chronic medication. Spontaneous remission is rare but can happen. Most treatment programs currently use a combination of stronger agents at first, which are then tapered down sometimes to a single agent as the disease responds. Many drugs may be taken safely for long periods of time, and they require a few months to produce a therapeutic response. Some, such as the nonsteroidal antiinflammatory drugs, work quickly and are most effective if taken every day. If effective, they may be taken on an "as needed" basis.

Why do I feel well on some days and terrible on others?

This is normal for most rheumatic diseases. Most rheumatic diseases fluctuate, seemingly independent of any obvious cause. Sometimes environmental factors such as weather may play a role.

If I can taper off my prednisone will my body go back to the way it was?

The typical moon face, upper back hump, and weight distribution that characterize chronic steroid use can resolve gradually after tapering off the medication. However, weight loss may not occur without diet and exercise.

Is exercise good for my joints?

No matter what type of arthritis you have, some form of exercise is not only good, but highly recommended. It is important to know that the stronger the tendons, ligaments, and muscles become, the more stable and protected your joint will be. However, some exercises, such as running on concrete or other hard surfaces, can be very traumatic for a particular joint. Pre-exercise stretching and warming up are very important to prevent injury. Water exercises are excellent for arthritis as a rule. In general, an exercise plan should be discussed with your rheumatologist and/or physical therapist.

Is there anything I can take for my fatigue?

Fatigue is a common complaint in patients with arthritis, and, like pain, does not necessarily correlate with joint destruction. While fatigue is a component of many chronic rheumatic diseases, it is important for rheumatologists to rule out other causes of fatigue, such as a sleep disorder, thyroid disorder, or psychological components caused by the arthritis. A regular exercise program can often help patients with chronic fatigue. There is some evidence that dehydroepiandrosterone (DHEA) might help decrease fatigue in lupus and possibly other rheumatic diseases. This point can be discussed with your rheumatologist.

What are the side effects of my medication?

Practically all medications have side effects. If you experience any unusual symptoms after starting a new medication, discuss it with your doctor.

Is there a cure for my arthritis?

There are no cures yet for most kinds of arthritis. However, we are getting better and better at controlling the symptoms of arthritis, and as medical science gains a better understanding of arthritis, it is reasonably to expect some types to be curable in the foreseeable future.

What kind of diet should I be on?

There really is no practical, specific diet for most kinds of arthritis. Gout is an exception, where foods high in purines should be avoided, that is, beans, sardines, anchovies, beer, and organ meats, such as kidney, brain, or pancreas. In general, though, a well-rounded diet low in saturated fats and high in fiber and fresh vegetables and fruit is excellent for general health.

Why am I so tired?

As a consequence of chronic inflammation, easy fatigability is a common complaint of patients with arthritis. Sometimes disturbed sleep is also a factor. Anti-inflammatory medication and medications that promote quality sleep, such as low dose amitriptyline, and cyclobenzaprine, can improve the problem.

Will physical therapy help?

Physical therapy and occupation therapy are very helpful for most patients with arthritis. Specific exercises taught by your practitioner might suffice. Proper exercises help prevent muscle atrophy and retard deformity.

Do you know of any support groups?

There are support groups for the various kinds of arthritis. Call your local Arthritis Foundation office, look in the local paper, or search the Internet for specific information.

Is this condition disabling?

Some people have such a severe case of arthritis that they will become disabled despite the advances in treatment. However, treatment is getting more effective all the time, and the future is encouraging.

Can you write a letter to my employer to modify my work environment?

Your practitioner can evaluate your specific case and write to your employer.

Does my medication need to be taken with food?

Some medications, such as aspirin, salsalate, and the other nonsteroidal anti-inflammatory drugs (ibuprofen, sulindac, naproxen, diclofenac, etc), are better tolerated if taken with food.

Which form of calcium should I take?

Calcium carbonate and calcium citrate are both readily absorbed. Calcium citrate is better if you take antacids, since the acid is necessary to absorb calcium carbonate. I encourage patients to obtain at least 50% of their daily calcium requirements from dietary calcium if possible.

How much calcium should I take?

The most important point is that daily-recommended doses are for elemental calcium. You must read labels to find out the amount of elemental calcium in the supplement. Calcium carbonate is 40% elemental calcium, thus 500mg of calcium carbonate is 200mg of elemental calcium. Calcium citrate is 20% elemental calcium; thus, 500 mg of calcium citrate is 100 mg elemental calcium. Recommendations for elemental calcium intake include 800 mg daily until age 10, and then 1200 mg daily during adolescence, and 1000 mg daily thereafter. During pregnancy and lactation, the recommended dose of elemental calcium is 1200 mg daily. For postmenopausal women not on estrogen replacement therapy, the recommended dose is 1500 mg daily.

What are the side effects of the medications for osteoporosis?

- **Alendronate** – GI irritation, especially esophageal; diarrhea, joint discomfort, and headache
- **Risedronate** – GI irritation, especially esophageal; diarrhea, joint discomfort, and headache
- **Calcitonin** – nasal spray – nasal irritation, rarely ulceration.
- **Raloxifene** – hot flashes, blood clots
- **Estrogen replacement therapy** – breast tenderness, vaginal bleeding, bloating, blood clots, breast cancer.

How often should I have bone mineral density testing?

This is individualized to the patient's situation. In general, while monitoring therapy, follow mineral densities testing every two years.

Are there any exercises that I can do to help my bones?

We recommend weigh-bearing exercises, if possible, such as walking. Exercise studies are very difficult to do to prove which exercises are the best. The greatest benefits of exercise are cardiovascular fitness, maintenance of strength, balance, muscle tone, and prevention of falls. Weight-bearing exercise does help maintain bone density.

Will estrogen replacement therapy (ERT) increase my risk of breast cancer?

There is evidence to support a small but significant increased risk of breast cancer in women who are on long term (>5 years) ERT.

Is my hip pain due to osteoporosis?

Most hip pain is due to arthritis, bursitis, or muscle problems. Osteoporosis causes pain from fractures of the soft bone. This pain is sudden and severe.

Do I also need magnesium with my calcium?

The otherwise healthy individual with a normal diet should not have magnesium deficiency. Unless there is evidence of magnesium depletion by appropriate testing, I do not recommend magnesium supplementation.

Should I avoid certain exercises that might predispose me to falling or breaking bones?

It is prudent for people with known osteoporosis to avoid major impact activities or those with a high potential for falling.

How much Vitamin D do I need to take to reduce my risk for fractures?

Recent data suggests that Vitamin D 800 IU daily is needed to significantly reduce the risk for both vertebral and non-vertebral fractures. It is also very important that anyone with a diagnosis of osteoporosis, especially a new diagnosis, have their vitamin D level checked by their physician.

For which alternative arthritis treatment is there some evidence of effectiveness (according to the Arthritis Foundation)?

- Glucosamine sulfate and chondroitin sulfate
- Cayenne (capsaicin)
- Evening primrose oil, barrage oil, fish oil
- Yoga, tai chi, qi gong
- Massage, meditation, hypnosis
- Acupuncture (perhaps)

REFERENCES

CHAPTER 1 – OSTEOARTHRITIS

1. Knowlton RG, Katzenstein PL, Moskowitz RW, Weaver EJ, Malemud CJ, Pathria MN, et al. Genetic linkage of a polymorphism in the type II procollagen gene (COL2A1) to primary osteoarthritis associated with mild chondrodysplasia. N Engl J Med 1990;322:526-30.
2. Belhorn LR, Hess EV. Erosive osteoarthritis. Seminars in Arthritis & Rheumatism 1993;22:298-306.
3. Bryant LR, des Rosier KF, Carpenter MT. Hydroxychloroquine in the treatment of erosive osteoarthritis. J Rheumatol 1995;22:1527-31.
4. Halverson PB, Carrera GF, McCarty DJ. Milwaukee shoulder syndrome. Fifteen additional cases and a description of contributing factors. Arch Intern Med 1990;150:677-82.
5. Utiger RD. Kashin-Beck disease--expanding the spectrum of iodine-deficiency disorders [editorial].N Engl J Med 1998;339:1156-8.
6. Agarwal SS, Phadke SR, Fredlund V,Viljoen D, Beighton P. Mseleni and Handigodu familial osteoarthropathies: syndromic identity? Am J Med Genet 1997;72:435-9.
7. Brandt K. Is a strong quadriceps muscle bad for a patient with knee osteoarthritis? (Editorial) Annals of Internal Medicine 2003;138:678-9.
8. Hinman RS, Bennell KL, Crossley KM, McConnell J. Immediate effects of adhesive tape on pain and disability in individuals with knee osteoarthritis. Rheumatology 2003;42:865-9.
9. Hochberg MC, Altman RD, Brandt KD, Clark BM, Dieppe PA,Griffin MR, et al. Guidelines for the medical management of osteoarthritis. Part I. Osteoarthritis of the hip. American College of Rheumatology. Arthritis & Rheumatism 1995;38:1535-40.
10. Hochberg MC, Altman RD, Brandt KD, Clark BM, Dieppe PA, Griffin MR, et al. Guidelines for the medical management of osteoarthritis. Part II. Osteoarthritis of the knee. American College of Rheumatology. Arthritis & Rheumatism 1995;38:1541-6.
11. Raynauld JP, Buckland-Wright C, Ward R, et al. Safety and efficacy of long-term intrarticular steroid injections in osteoarthritis of the knee: a randomized, double-blind, placebo-controlled trial. Arthritis Rheum 2003:48:370-7.
12. Emkey R, Rosenthal N, Wu SC, Jordan D, Kamin M. Efficacy and safety of tramadol/acetaminophen tablets as add-on therapy for osteoarthritis pain in subjects receiving a COX-2 nonsteroidal antiinflammatory drug: a multicenter, randomized, double-blind, placebo-controlled trial. J Rheumatol 2004; 31:150-6.
13. Tubach F, Ravaud R, Baron G, et al. Evaluation of clinically relevant states in patient reported outcomes in knee and hip osteoarthritis: the patient acceptable symptom state. Ann Rheum Dis 2005;64:34-7.
14. Bijlsma JWJ. Patient centered outcomes in osteoarthritis. Ann Rheum Dis 2005;64:1-2.
15. Brandt KD, Mazzuca SA. Lessons learned from nine clinical trials of disease-modifying osteoarthritis drugs. Arthritis Rheum 2005;52:3349-59.
16. Cole AA, Chubinskaya S, Luchene LJ, Chlebek K, Orth MW, Greenwald RA, et al. Doxycycline disrupts chondrocyte differentiation and inhibits cartilage matrix degradation. Arthritis & Rheumatism 1994;37:1727-34.

CHAPTER 2 – OSTEOPOROSIS

1. Chrischilles EA, Butler CD, Davis CS, Wallace RB, A model of lifetime osteoporosis impact. Arch Intern. Med 1991;151(10):2026-32.
2. Americas Bone Health: The State of Osteoporosis and Low Bone Mass in our Nation NOF 2002.
3. National Osteoporosis Foundation Osteop Int 1998,8:S1-S88.
4. Kado DM, Browner WS, Palermo L, Nevitt MC, Genant HK, Cummings SR, Vertebral fractures and mortality in older women: a prospective study. Study of Osteoporotic Fractures Research Group Arch Int Med 1999;159(11):1215-1226.
5. Ray NF, Chan JK, Thamer M, Melton LJ 3rd. Medical expenditures for the treatment of osteoporotic fractures in the United States in 1995: report from the National Osteoporosis Foundation J Bone Miner Res 1997;12(1):24-35.
6. Forsen L, Sogaard AJ, Meyer HE, Edna T, Kopjar B. Survival after hip fracture: short and long-term excess mortality according to age and gender Osteop Int 1999; 10(1)73-7.
7. Gluer CC,Cummings SR,Pressman A, Li J, Gluer K,Faulkner KG, et al. Prediction of hip fractures from pelvic radiographs: the study of osteoporotic fractures. The Study of Osteoporotic Fractures Research Group. Journal of Bone & Mineral Research 1994;9(5):671-7.
8. Faulkner KG,McClung M,Cummings SR.Automated evaluation of hip axis length for predicting hip fracture. Journal of Bone & Mineral Research 1994;9(7):1065-70.
9. Reid IR, Chin K,Evans MC, Jones JG. Relation between increase in length of hip axis in older women between 1950s and 1990s and increase in age specific rates of hip fracture [see comments]. Br Med J 1994;309(6953):508-9.
10. Faulkner KG,McClung M,Cummings SR.Automated evaluation of hip axis length for predicting hip fracture. Journal of Bone & Mineral Research 1994;9(7):1065-70.
11. Reid IR, Chin K,Evans MC, Jones JG. Relation between increase in length of hip axis in older women between 1950s and 1990s and increase in age specific rates of hip fracture [see comments]. Br Med J 1994;309(6953):508-9.
12. Hayes WC,Piazza SJ, Zysset PK.Biomechanics of fracture risk prediction of the hip and spine by quantitative computed tomography. Radiol Clin North Am 1991;29(1):1-18.
13. Genant HK, Gluer CC, Lotz JC. Gender differences in bone density, skeletal geometry, and fracture biomechanics [editorial;comment].Radiology 1994;190(3):636-40.
14. Mazess RB.Fracture risk: a role for compact bone [editorial] [see comments]. Calcif Tissue Int 1990;47(4):191-3.
15. Rozenberg S,Vandromme J,Kroll M, Praet JP,Peretz A,Ham H.Overview of the clinical usefulness of bone mineral measurements in the prevention of postmenopausal osteoporosis. International Journal of Fertility & Menopausal Studies 1995;40(1):12-24.
16. Wasnich RD. Epidemiology of osteoporosis. In:Favus,MJ, ed. Primer on the Metabolic Bone Diseases and Disorders of Mineral Metabolism, 4th ed. Philadelphia PA: Lippincott,Williams and Wilkins 1999; 257-9.
17. Anonymous.Assessment of fracture risk and its application to screening for postmenopausal osteoporosis.Report of a WHO Study Group.World Health Organ Tech Rep Ser 1994;843:1-129.
18. Melton LJ, Riggs BL: Epidemiology of age-related fractures. In:Avioli LV ed.The Osteoporotic Syndrome:Detection, prevention and treatment.New York:Grune and Stratton 1983; 45-72.
19. Solomon L. Osteoporosis and fracture of the femoral neck in the South African Bantu. Journal of Bone & Joint Surgery -British Volume 1968;50(1):2-13.

20. Ross PD,Norimatsu H, Davis JW,Yano K,Wasnich RD, Fujiwara S, et al.A comparison of hip fracture incidence among native Japanese, Japanese Americans, and American Caucasians.Am J Epidemiol 1991;133(8):801-9.

21. Marcus R.Physical activity and regulation of bone mass. In:Favus MJ ed. Primer on the Metabolic Bone Diseases and Disorders of Mineral Metabolism, 4th ed. Philadelphia PA: Lippincott,Williams and Wilkins 1999; 262-4.

22. Snow-Harter C, Marcus R. Exercise, bone mineral density, and osteoporosis. Exercise & Sport Sciences Reviews 1991;19:351-88.

23. Slemenda CW, Miller JZ, Hui SL, Reister TK,Johnston CC, Jr. Role of physical activity in the development of skeletal mass in children. Journal of Bone & Mineral Research 1991;6(11):1227-33.

24. Ruiz JC, Mandel C,Garabedian M. Influence of spontaneous calcium intake and physical exercise on the vertebral and femoral bone mineral density of children and adolescents. Journal of Bone & Mineral Research 1995;10(5):675-82.

25. Recker RR, Davies KM, Hinders SM,Heaney RP,Stegman MR,Kimmel DB.Bone gain in young adult women [see comments].JAMA 1992;268(17):2403-8.

26. Simkin A,Ayalon J, Leichter I. Increased trabecular bone density due to bone-loading exercises in postmenopausal osteoporotic women.Calcif Tissue Int 1987;40(2):59-63.

27. Dalsky GP, Stocke KS, Ehsani AA, Slatopolsky E, Lee WC,Birge SJ, Jr.Weight-bearing exercise training and lumbar bone mineral content in postmenopausal women.Ann Intern Med 1988;108(6):824-8.

28. Menkes A, Mazel S,Redmond RA,Koffler K, Libanati CR,Gundberg CM,et al. Strength training increases regional bone mineral density and bone remodeling in middle-aged and older men. J Appl Physiol 1993;74(5):2478-84.

29. Notelovitz M,Martin D,Tesar R,Khan FY,Probart C,Fields C, et al. Estrogen therapy and variable-resistance weight training increase bone mineral in surgically menopausal women [see comments]. Journal of Bone & Mineral Research 1991;6(6):583-90.

30. Cummings SR,Nevitt MC, Browner WS,Stone K,Fox KM,Ensrud KE, et al. Risk factors for hip fracture in white women. Study of Osteoporotic Fractures Research Group [see comments]. N Engl J Med 1995;332(12):767-73.

31. Spector TD,Hall GM,McCloskey EV, Kanis JA. Risk of vertebral fracture in women with rheumatoid arthritis. Br Med J 1993;306(6877):558.

32. Hooyman JR, Melton LJd, Nelson AM,O'Fallon WM,Riggs BL.Fractures after rheumatoid arthritis. A population-based study.Arthritis & Rheumatism 1984;27(12):1353-61.

33. Michel BA, Bloch DA,Fries JF.Predictors of fractures in early rheumatoid arthritis. J Rheumatol 1991;18(6):804-8.

34. Verstraeten A, Dequeker J.Vertebral and peripheral bone mineral content and fracture incidence in postmenopausal patients with rheumatoid arthritis: effect of low dose corticosteroids. Ann Rheum Dis 1986;45(10):852-7.

35. Jergas M,Genant HK.Current methods and recent advances in the diagnosis of osteoporosis. Arthritis & Rheumatism 1993;36(12):1649-62.

36. Dawson-Hughes B, Harris SS,Krall EA, Dallal GE. Effect of calcium and vitamin D supplementation on bone density in men and women 65 years of age or older [see comments]. N Engl J Med 1997;337(10):670-6.

37. Lindsay R. Sex steroids in the pathogenesis and prevention of osteoporosis. In: Riggs BL ed. Osteoporosis: Etiology, diagnosis and management.New York:Raven Press 1988; 333-58.

38. Kiel DP,Felson DT,Anderson JJ,Wilson PW,Moskowitz MA. Hip fracture and the use of estrogens in postmenopausal women.The Framingham Study. N Engl J Med 1987;317(19):1169-74.

39. Cauley JA, Seeley DG, Ensrud K, Ettinger B, Black D,Cummings SR.Estrogen replacement therapy and fractures in older women.Study of Osteoporotic Fractures Research Group.Ann Intern Med 1995;122(1):9-16.

40. Lindsay R, Hart DM, Clark DM.The minimum effective dose of estrogen for prevention of postmenopausal bone loss. Obstetrics & Gynecology 1984;63(6):759-63.

41. Ettinger B, Black DM,Mitlak BH,Knickerbocker RK, Nickelsen T,Genant HK,et al. Reduction of vertebral fracture risk in postmenopausal women with osteoporosis treated with raloxifene: results from a 3-year randomized clinical trial. Multiple Outcomes of Raloxifene Evaluation (MORE) Investigators [see comments] [published erratum appears in JAMA 1999 Dec 8;282(22):2124]. JAMA 1999;282(7):637-45.

42. Delmas PD, Bjarnason NH, Mitlak BH,Ravoux AC, Shah AS, Huster WJ, et al. Effects of raloxifene on bone mineral density, serum cholesterol concentrations, and uterine endometrium in postmenopausal women [see comments]. N Engl J Med 1997;337(23):1641-7.

43. McClung M,Clemmesen B,Daifotis A, Gilchrist NL, Eisman J,Weinstein RS, et al. Alendronate prevents postmenopausal bone loss in women without osteoporosis.A double-blind, randomized, controlled trial.Alendronate Osteoporosis Prevention Study Group [see comments]. Ann Intern Med 1998;128(4):253-61.

44. Harris ST,Watts NB,Genant HK,McKeever CD,Hangartner T,Keller M, et al. Effects of risedronate treatment on vertebral and nonvertebral fractures in women with postmenopausal osteoporosis: a randomized controlled trial.Vertebral Efficacy With Risedronate Therapy (VERT) Study Group [see comments]. JAMA 1999;282(14):1344-52.

45. Mortensen L, Charles P, Bekker PJ, Digennaro J, Johnston CC, Jr. Risedronate increases bone mass in an early postmenopausal population:two years of treatment plus one year of follow-up. Journal of Clinical Endocrinology & Metabolism 1998;83(2):396-402.

46. Reginster YP, Adami S, Lakatos P, et al. Efficacy and tolerability of once-monthly oral ibandronate in postmenopausal osteoporosis: 2 year results from the MOBILE study. Annals of Rheumatic Diseases 2006; 65:654-61

47. Overgaard K,Hansen MA,Jensen SB,Christiansen C. Effect of salcatonin given intranasally on bone mass and fracture rates in established osteoporosis: a dose-response study. Br Med J 1992;305(6853):556-61.

48. Neer RM, Arnaud CD, Zanchetta JR, Prince R, Gaich GA, et al Effect of parathyroid hormone(1-34) on fracture and bone mineral density in postmenopausal women with osteoporosis N Engl J Med 2001; 344: 1434-41.

CHAPTER 3 – PAGET'S DISEASE OF BONE

1. Lash R: Paget's disease. In: Klippel JH (ed): Primer on the Rheumatic Diseases, 12th ed., 2001. Atlanta, The Arthritis Foundation, p 508-509.

2. Hines SE. Paget's disease of bone: a new philosophy of treatment. Patient Care 1999;33:40-60.

3. Cooper C, Dennison E, Schafheutle k, et al. Epidemiology of Paget's disease of bone. Bone 1999;24:S3-S5.

CHAPTER 4 – OSTEONECROSIS

1. Alarcon GS: Osteonecrosis. In: Klippel JH (ed): Primer on the Rheumatic Diseases, 12th ed., 2001. Atlanta, The Arthritis Foundation, p 503-506.
2. Arlet J, Ficat P. Diagnostic de l'osteonecrose femorocapitale primitive au stade I (stade preradiologic): [The diagnosis of primary femur head osteonecrosis at stage I (pre-radiologic stage)]. Rev Chir Orthop Reparatrice Appar Mot 1968;54:637-648.
3. Urbaniak JR, Coogan PG, Gunneson EB, Nunley JA. Treatment of osteonecrosis of the femoral head with free vascularized fibular grafting. A long-term follow-up study of one hundred and three hips. J Bone Joint Surg Am 1995;77:681-94.

CHAPTER 5 – FIBROMYALGIA

1. Goldenberg DL. Update on the treatment of fibromyalgia. Bulletin on the Rheumatic Diseases 2004;53:1-7.
2. Hadler NM. "Fibromyalgia" and the medicalization of misery. J Rheumatol 2003;30:1668-70.
3. Wallace DJ, Shapiro S,Panush RS. Update on fibromyalgia syndrome.Bull Rheum Dis 1999;48:1-4.
4. Wolfe F,Anderson J. Silicone filled breast implants and the risk of fibromyalgia and rheumatoid arthritis [published erratum appears in J Rheumatol 2000 Mar;27(3):825]. J Rheumatol 1999;26:2025-8.
5. Lai S, Goldman JA, Child AH, Engel A, Lamm SH. Fibromyalgia, hypermobility, and breast implants. J Rheumatol 2000;27:2237-41.
6. Hadhazy V, Ezzo JM, Berman, BM, et al. Mind and body therapy for fibromyalgia. Cochrane Database Syst Rev 2003; 3.
7. Mannerkorpi K, Ahlmen M, Ekdahl C. Six- and 24-month follow-up of pool exercise therapy and education for patients with fibromyalgia. Scand J Rheumatol 2002;31:306-10.
8. Burckhardt CS, Bjelle A. Education programmes for fibromyalgia patients: Description and evaluation. Baillieres Clin Rheumatol 1994;8:935-55.
9. Arnold LM, Hess EV, Hudson JL, et al. A randomized, placebo-controlled, double-blind, flexible-dose study of fluoxetine in the treatment of woman with fibromyalgia. Amer J Med 2002;112:191-7.
10. Bennet RM, Kamin M, Karin R, Rosenthal N. Tramadol and acetaminophen combination tablets in the treatment of fibromyalgia pain: a double-blind, randomized, placebo-controlled study. Am J Med 2003;114:537-45.

CHAPTER 6 – THE AMYLOIDOSES

1. Westermark P, Benson MD, Buxbaum JN, et al. Amyloid fibril protein nomenclature - 2002. Amyloid 2002;9:197-200.
2. Hayman SR. Lacy MQ. Kyle RA. Gertz MA. Primary systemic amyloidosis: a cause of malabsorption syndrome. American Journal of Medicine. 2001;111:535-40.

3. Diaz RJ, Washburn S, Cauble L, et al. The effect of dialyzer reprocessing on performance and beta2-microglobulin removal using polysulfone membranes. American Journal of Kidney Disease 1993;21:405-10
4. Raj DS, Ouwendyk M, Francoeur R, Pierratos A. beta(2)-microglobulin kinetics in nocturnal haemodialysis. Nephrol Dial Transplant 2000;15:58-64.
5. Buxbaum JN, Tagoe CE. The genetics of the amyloidoses. Annu Rev Med 2000;51:543-69.
6. Jacobson DR, Pastore RD, Yaghoubian R, et al. Variant-sequence transthyretin (isoleucine 122) in late-onset cardiac amyloidosis in Black Americans. N Engl J Med 1997;336:466-73.
7. Merlini G, Belloti,V. Mechanisms of disease: Molecular mechanisms of amyloidosis. New Engl J Med 2003;349:583-96.
8. Skinner M; Sanchorawala V; Seldin DC; High-dose melphalan and autologous stem-cell transplantation in patients with AL amyloidosis: an 8-year study. Ann Intern Med 2004;40:85-93.

CHAPTER 7 – RHEUMATOID ARTHRITIS

1. Arnett FC, Edworthy SM, Bloch DA, McShane DJ, Fries JF, Cooper NS, et al. The American Rheumatism Association 1987 revised criteria for the classification of rheumatoid arthritis. Arthritis & Rheumatism 1988;31:315-24.
2. van Zeben D, Breedveld FC. Prognostic factors in rheumatoid arthritis. Journal of Rheumatology - Supplement 1996;44:31-3.
3. Lee DM, Shur PH. Clinical utility of the anti-CCP assay in patients with rheumatic diseases. Annals of the Rheumatic Diseases 2003;62:870-4.
4. Ehrenfeld M, Gur H, Shoenfeld Y. Rheumatologic features of hematologic disorders. Curr Opin Rheumatol 1999;11:62-7.
5. Fautrel B, LeMoel G, Siant-Marcoux B, et al. Diagnostic value of ferritin and glycosylated ferritin in adult onset Still's disease. Journal of Rheumatology 2001;28: 322-9.
6. Lambert CM, Sandhu S, Lochhead A, Hurst NP, McRorie E, Dhillon V. Dose escalation of parenteral methotrexate in active rheumatoid arthritis that has been unresponsive to conventional doses of methotrexate: a randomized, controlled trial. Arthritis Rheum 2004;50:364-71.
7. Taylor PC. Anti-tumor necrosis factor therapies. Current Opinion in Rheumatology 2001;13:164-9.
8. Olsen NJ, Stein CM. Drug Therapy: new drugs for rheumatoid arthritis. N Engl J Med 2004;350:2167-79.
9. O'Dell JR.. Drug therapy: therapeutic strategies for rheumatoid arthritis. N Engl J Med 2004;350:2591-602.
10. American College of Rheumatology Subcommittee on Rheumatoid Arthritis Guidelines. Guidelines for the management of rheumatoid arthritis: 2002 Update. Arthritis & Rheum 2002;46:328-46.
11. Case JP. Old and new drugs used in rheumatoid arthritis: a historical perspective. Part 2: the newer drugs and drug strategies. American Journal of Therapeutics 2001;8:163-79.
12. Kremer JM, Westhovens R, Leon M, et al. Treatment of rheumatoid arthritis by selective inhibition of T-cell activation with fusion protein CTLA4Ig. N Engl J Med 2003; 349:1907-15.
13. Edwards JCW, Szczepanski L, Szechinski J, et al. Efficacy and safety of rituximab, a B cell targeted chimeric monoclonal antibody: a placebo RCT in patients with RA. Arthritis Rheum 2002;46:S197.

14. Gottenberg JE, Guillevin L, Lambotte O, et al. Tolerance and short-term efficacy of rituximab in 43 patients with systemic autoimmune diseases. Ann Rheum Dis 2004;DOI:10.1135/ard2004.029694.
15. Elliott JR, Paulsen GA, Mallek JA, et al. Treatment of early sero-positive rheumatoid arthritis: doxycycline versus methotrexate alone (abstract). Arthritis Rheum 2003;48:S654.
16. Stone M, Fortin PR, Pacheco-Tena C, Inman RD. Should tetracycline treatment be used more extensively for rheumatoid arthritis? Meta-analysis demonstrates clinical benefit with reduction in disease activity. J Rheumatol 2003;30:2112-22.
17. Pincus T, Summey JA, Soraci SA Jr.,Wallston KA, Hummon NP. Assessment of patient satisfaction in activities of daily living using a modified Stanford Health Assessment Questionnaire. Arthritis & Rheumatism 1983;26:1346-53.
18. Callahan LF, Pincus T, Huston JW 3rd, Brooks RH, Nance EP Jr., Kaye JJ. Measures of activity and damage in rheumatoid arthritis: depiction of changes and prediction of mortality over five years. Arthritis Care & Research 1997;10:381-94.
19. Goekoop-Ruiterman YP, de Vries-Bouwstra JK, Allaart CF, et al. Clinical and radiographic outcomes of four different treatment strategies on patients with early rheumatoid arthritis (the BeSt study): a randomized, controlled trial. Arthritis Rheum 2005;52:3381-90.
20. Breedveld FC, Weisman MH, Kavanaugh AF, et al. The PREMIER study. Arthritis Rheum 2006;54:26-37.

CHAPTER 8 – SYSTEMIC LUPUS ERYTHEMATOSUS

1. Weening JJ, D'Agati VD, Schwartz MM, et al. The classification of glomerulonephritis in systemic lupus erythematosus revisited. Kidney Int 2004;65:521-30.
2. Tan EM, Cohen AS, Fries JF, Masi AT, McShane DJ, Rothfield NF, et al. The 1982 revised criteria for the classification of systemic lupus erythematosus. Arthritis & Rheumatism 1982;25:1271-7.
3. Tan EM. Antinuclear antibodies: diagnostic markers for autoimmune diseases and probes for cell biology. Adv Immunol 1989;44:93-151.
4. Tsakonas E, Joseph L, Esdaile JM, et al. A long-term study of hydroxychloroquine withdrawal on exacerbations in systemic lupus erythematosus. The Canadian Hydroxychloroquine Study Group. Lupus 1998;7:80-5.

5. Contreras G, Pardo V, Leclercq B, Lenz O, Tozman E, O'Nan P, Roth D. Sequential therapies for proliferative lupus nephritis. N Engl J Med 2004; 350:971-80.)

6. Gescuk BD, Davis JC Jr. Novel therapeutic agents for systemic lupus erythematosus. Current Opinion in Rheumatology 2002;14:515-21.
7. Looney RJ, Anolik J, Sanz I. Treatment of SLE with anti-CD20 monoclonal antibody. Current Directions in Autoimmunity 2005;8:193-205.
8. Pisoni CN, Sanchez FJ, Karim Y, et el. Mycophenolate mofetil in systemic lupus erythematosus : efficacy and tolerability in 86 patients. J Rheum 2005;32:1047-52
9. Urowitz MB, Gladman DD. Rheumatic disease in pregnancy. In: Burrow GN, Ferris TF eds. Medical complications during pregnancy, 3rd ed. Philadelphia PA: W.B. Saunders Company 1988; 499-525.
10. Petri M. Pregnancy in SLE. Baillieres Clin Rheumatol 1998;12:449-76.
11. Buyon JP. Hormone replacement therapy in postmenopausal women with systemic lupus erythematosus. J Am Med Womens Assoc 1998;53:13-7.

12. Roman MJ, Shanker BA, Davis A, et al. Prevalence and correlates of accelerated atherosclerosis in systemic lupus erythematosus. N Eng J Med 2003:349:2399-406.

13. Asanuma Y, Oeser A, Shintani AK, et al. Premature coronary-artery atherosclerosis in systemic lupus erythematosus. N Engl J Med 2003;349:2407-15.

CHAPTER 9 – ANTIPHOSPHOLIPID SYNDROME

1. McNeil HP, Chesterman CN, Krilis SA. Immunology and clinical importance of antiphospholipid antibodies. Adv Immunol 1991;49:193-280.

2. Wilson WA, Gharavi AE. Hughes syndrome: perspectives on thrombosis and antiphospholipid antibody [editorial].Am J Med 1996;101:574-5.

3. Schulman S, Svenungsson E, Granqvist S. Anticardiolipin antibodies predict early recurrence of thromboembolism and death among patients with venous thromboembolism following anticoagulant therapy. Duration of Anticoagulation Study Group. American Journal of Medicine 1998;104:332-8

4. Khamashta MA, Cuadrado MJ, Mujic F, et al. The management of thrombosis in the antiphospholipid-antibody syndrome. New England Journal of Medicine 1995;332:993-7.

5. Cuadrado MJ. Treatment and monitoring of patients with antiphospholipid antibodies and thrombotic history (Hughes syndrome). Curr Rheumatol Rep 2002;4:392-8.

6. Crowther MA, Ginsberg JS, Julian J, et al. A comparison of two intensities or warfarin for the prevention of recurrent thrombosis in patients with the antiphospholipid antibody syndrome. N Engl J Med 2003;349;1133-1138.

7. Levine SR, Brey RL, Tilley BC, et al. Antiphospholipid antibodies and subsequent thrombo-occlusive events in patients with ischemic stroke. JAMA 2004;291:576-84.

8. Hylek EM, Heiman H, Skates SJ, et al. Acetaminophen and other risk factors for excessive warfarin anticoagulation. JAMA 1998;279:657-62.

9. Watzke HH, Forberg E, Svolba G, et al. A prospective controlled trial comparing weekly self-testing and self-dosing with the standard management of patients on stable oral anticoagulation. Thomb Haemost 2000;83:661-5.

10. Cowchock S. Treatment of antiphospholipid syndrome in pregnancy. Lupus 1998;7(Suppl 2):S95-7.

11. Triolo G, Ferrante A, Ciccia F, et al. Randomized study of subcutaneous low molecular weight heparin plus aspirin versus intravenous immune globulin in the treatment of recurrent fetal loss associated with antiphospholipid antibodies. Arthritis Rheum 2003;48:728-31.

12. Petri M. Pathogenesis and treatment of the antiphospholipid antibody syndrome. Medical Clinics of North America 1997;81:151-77.

CHAPTER 10 – SJÖGREN'S SYNDROME

1. Fox RI. Clinical features, pathogenesis, and treatment of Sjogren's syndrome. Curr Opin Rheumatol 1996;8:438-45.

2. Carsons S, Talal N. Sjögren's syndrome in the 21st century. International Journal of Advances in Rheumatology 2003;1:139-7.

3. Classification criteria for Sjogren's syndrome: a revised version of the European criteria proposed by the American-European Consensus Group. Annals of the Rheumatic Diseases 2002;61:554-8.

4. Kong L, Ogawa N, Nakabayashi T, et al. Fas and Fas-ligand expression in the salivary glands of patients with primary Sjögren's syndrome. Arthritis & Rheumatism 40:87-97, 1997.

5. Sun D, Emmert-Buck MR, Fox PC. Differential cytokine mRNA expression in human labial minor salivary glands in primary Sjögren's syndrome. Autoimmunity 1998;28:125-37.

6. Williams FM,Cohen PR,Jumshyd J,Reveille JD.Prevalence of the diffuse infiltrative lymphocytosis syndrome among human immunodeficiency virus type 1-positive outpatients. Arthritis & Rheumatism 1998;41:863-8.

7. Boki KA, Iannidis JP, Segas JV, et al. How significant is sensorineural hearing loss in primary Sjögren's syndrome? Journal of Rheumatology 2001;28:798-801.

8. Fox RI, Saito I. Criteria for diagnosis of Sjogren's syndrome. Rheum Dis Clin North Am 1994;20:391-407.

9. Schrot RJ, Adelman HM, Linden CN, Wallach PM. Cystic parotid gland enlargement in HIV disease. The diffuse infiltrative lymphocytosis syndrome. JAMA 1997;278:166-7.

10. Lee M, Rutka JA, Slomovic AR, et al. Establishing guidelines for the role of minor salivary gland biopsy in clinical practice for Sjögren's syndrome. Journal of Rheumatology 1998;25:247-53.

11. Diss TC, Wotherspoon AC, Speight P, Pan L, Isaacson PG. B-cell monoclonality, Epstein Barr virus, and t(14;18) in myoepithelial sialadenitis and low-grade B-cell MALT lymphoma of the parotid gland. Am J Surg Pathol 1995;19:531-6.

12. Vivino FB, Al-Hashimi I, Khan Z, LeVeque FG, Salisbury PL, 3rd, Tran-Johnson TK, et al. Pilocarpine tablets for the treatment of dry mouth and dry eye symptoms in patients with Sjogren syndrome: a randomized, placebo-controlled, fixed-dose, multicenter trial. P92-01 Study Group. Arch Intern Med 1999;159:174-81.

13. Steinfeld SD, Demols P, Appelboom T. Infliximab in primary Sjögren's syndrome. Arthritis & Rheumatism 2002;46:3301-3.

14. Ioannidis JP, Vassiliou VA, Moutsopoulos HM. Long-term risk of mortality and lymphoproliferative disease and predictive classification of primary Sjogren's syndrome. Arthritis Rheum 2002; 46:741–7.

CHAPTER 11 – IDIOPATHIC INFLAMMATORY MYOPATHIES

1. Bohan A, Peter JB, Bowman RL ,Pearson CM. Computer-assisted analysis of 153 patients with polymyositis and dermatomyositis. Medicine 1977;56:255-86.

2. Plotz PH, Dalakas M, Leff RL, Love LA, Miller FW, Cronin ME. Current concepts in the idiopathic inflammatory myopathies: polymyositis, dermatomyositis, and related disorders. Ann Intern Med 1989;111:143-57.

3. Hengstman GJ, van Engelen BG, Vree Egberts WT, van Venrooij WJ. Myositis-specific autoantibodies: overview and recent developments. Current opinion in Rheumatology 2001;13:476-82.

4. Oddis CV. Therapy of inflammatory myopathy. Rheum Dis Clin North Am 1994;20:899-918.

5. Plotz PH, Rider LG, Targoff IN, Raben N, O'Hanlon TP, Miller FW. NIH conference. Myositis: immunologic contributions to understanding cause, pathogenesis, and therapy. Ann Intern Med 1995;122:715-24.

6. Dalakas MC. Clinical benefits and immunopathological correlates of intravenous immune globulin in the treatment of inflammatory myopathies. Clinical & Experimental Immunology 1996;104(Suppl 1):55-60.

CHAPTER 12 – SYSTEMIC SCLEROSIS (SCLERODERMA)

1. Polisson RP, Anderson PA, Gilkeson G, Harris N, Kay J, Khan M, Manzi, Simms R, Simon L: Scleroderma and inflammatory myopathies. In: Rheumatology medical knowledge self-assessment program, 11th ed. Philadelphia PA: American College of Physicians 1997; 169-82.
2. LeRoy EC. A brief overview of the pathogenesis of scleroderma (systemic sclerosis). Ann Rheum Dis 1992;51:286-8.
3. Silman AJ. Scleroderma. Baillieres Clin Rheumatol 1995:471-82.
4. Steen VD, Powell DL, Medsger TA, Jr. Clinical correlations and prognosis based on serum autoantibodies in patients with systemic sclerosis. Arthritis & Rheumatism 1988;31:196-203.
5. Iooannidis JPA, Vvlachoyiannopoulis PG, Haidich A-B, et al. Mortality in systemic sclerosis: an international meta-analysis of individual patient data. Am J Med 2005;118:2-10.
6. Kahaleh MB. Endothelin, an endothelial-dependent vasoconstrictor in scleroderma. Enhanced production and profibrotic action. Arthritis Rheum 1991; 34:978-83.
7. Nelson, JL. Microchimerism and autoimmune disease [editorial]. N Engl J Med 1998;338:1224.) In this vein, Graft versus host disease has several of the features of systemic sclerosis
8. Steen VD, Costantino JP, Shapiro AP, Medsger TA, Jr. Outcome of renal crisis in systemic sclerosis: relation to availability of angiotensin converting enzyme (ACE) inhibitors. Ann Intern Med 1990;113:352-7.
9. Steen VD, Medsger TA, Jr., Rodnan GP. D-Penicillamine therapy in progressive systemic sclerosis (scleroderma): a retrospective analysis. Ann Intern Med 1982;97:652-9.
10. Martinez FJ, McCune WJ. Cyclophosphamide for scleroderma lung disease. (Editorial) N Eng J Med 2006;354:2707-08.

CHAPTER 13 – THE MIXED CONNECTIVE TISSUE DISEASE

1. Lehman TJA: Connective tissue disease and non-articular rheumatism. In: Klippel J,Weyand CM, Wortmann RL eds. Primer on the Rheumatic Diseases, 11th ed. Atlanta GA: The Arthritis Foundation 1997; 398-403.
2. Kasukawa R, Tojo T, Miyawaki S. Preliminary diagnostic criteria for classification of mixed connective tissue disease. In: Kasukawa R, Sharp GC eds. Mixed connective tissue disease and anti nuclear antibodies. Amsterdam:Elsevier; 1987: 41-7.
3. Burdt MA, Hoffman RW, Deutscher SL, Wang GS, Johnson JC, Sharp GC. Long-term outcome in mixed connective tissue disease: longitudinal clinical and serologic findings. Arthritis & Rheumatism 1999;42:899-909.
4. Mairesse N, Kahn MF, Appelboom T. Antibodies to the constitutive 73-kd heat shock protein: a new marker of mixed connective tissue disease? Am J Med 1993;95:595-00.

CHAPTER 14 – GIANT CELL ARTERITIS AND POLYMYALGIA RHEUMATICA

1. Salvarani C, Gabriel SE, O'Fallon WM, Hunder GG. The incidence of giant cell arteritis in Olmsted County, Minnesota: apparent fluctuations in a cyclic pattern. Ann Intern Med 1995;123:192-4.
2. Salvarani C, Macchioni PL, Tartoni PL, Rossi F, Baricchi R, Castri C, et al. Polymyalgia rheumatica and giant cell arteritis: a 5-year epidemiologic and clinical study in Reggio Emilia, Italy. Clinical & Experimental Rheumatology 1987;5:205-15.
3. Friedman G, Friedman B, Benbassat J. Epidemiology of temporal arteritis in Israel. Isr J Med Sci 1982;18:241-4.
4. Weyand CM, Hicok KC, Hunder GG, Goronzy JJ. Tissue cytokine patterns in patients with polymyalgia rheumatica and giant cell arteritis. Ann Intern Med 1994;121:484-91.
5. Weyand CM, Tetzlaff N, Bjornsson J, Brack A,Younge B, Goronzy JJ. Disease patterns and tissue cytokine profiles in giant cell arteritis. Arthritis & Rheumatism 1997;40:19-26.
6. Hunder GC: Vasculitis. In: Klippel J, Weyand CM, Wortmann RL eds. Primer on the Rheumatic Diseases, 11th ed.Atlanta GA: The Arthritis Foundation 1997; 289-300.
7. Nuenninghoff DM, Hudner GG, Christianson TJ, et al. Incidence and predictors of large-artery complication (aortic aneurysm, aortic dissection, and/or large-artery stenosis) in patients with giant cell arteritis: a population–based study over 50 years. Arthritis Rheum 2003:48:3522-31.
8. Hellmann DB. Update in Rheumatology. Ann Intern Med 2004;141:801-4.
9. Gordon LK, Levin LA. Visual loss in giant cell arteritis. JAMA 1998;280:385-6.
10. Swannell AJ. Polymyalgia rheumatica and temporal arteritis: diagnosis and management. Br Med J 1997;314(7090):1329-32.
11. Ghanchi FD, Dutton GN. Current concepts in giant cell (temporal) arteritis. Surv Ophthalmol 1997;42:99-123.
12. Hayreh SS, Podhajsky PA, Raman R, Zimmerman B. Giant cell arteritis: validity and reliability of various diagnostic criteria. Am J Ophthalmol 1997;123:285-96.
13. Achkar AA, Lie JT, Hunder GG, O'Fallon WM,Gabriel SE. How does previous corticosteroid treatment affect the biopsy findings in giant cell (temporal) arteritis? Ann Intern Med 1994;120:987-92.
14. Myklebust G, Gran JT. A prospective study of 287 patients with polymyalgia rheumatica and temporal arteritis: clinical and laboratory manifestations at onset of disease and at the time of diagnosis. Br J Rheumatol 1996;35:1161-8.
15. Nesher G, Berkun Y, Mates M, Baras M, Rubinow A, Sonnenblick M. Low-dose aspirin and prevention of cranial ischemic complications in giant cell arteritis. Arthritis Rheum 2004;50:1332-7.

CHAPTER 15 – OTHER VASCULITIDES

1. Watts RA, Lane SE, Bentham G, Scott DG. Epidemiology of systemic vasculitis: a ten-year study in the United Kingdom. Arthritis & Rheumatism 2000;43:414-9.
2. Watts RA, Scott DG. Classification and epidemiology of the vasculitides. Baillieres Clin Rheumatol 1997;11:191-217.

3. Watts RA. Scott DG. Epidemiology of the vasculitides. Current Opinion in Rheumatology 2003;15:11-6.
4. Leavitt RY, Fauci AS. Less common manifestations and presentations of Wegener's granulomatosis. Curr Opin Rheumatol 1992;4:16-22.
5. Hoffman GS. Classification of the systemic vasculitides: antineutrophil cytoplasmic antibodies, consensus and controversy [editorial]. Clinical & Experimental Rheumatology 1998;16:111-5.
6. Lhote F, Guillevin L. Polyarteritis nodosa, microscopic polyangiitis, and Churg-Strauss syndrome. Clinical aspects and treatment. Rheum Dis Clin North Am 1995;21:911-47.
7. Lamprecht P, Gause A, Gross WL. Cryoglobulinemic vasculitis. Arthritis & Rheumatism 1999; 42:2507-16.
8. Hoffman GS, Kerr GS, Leavitt RY, Hallahan CW, Lebovics RS, Travis WD, et al. Wegener granulomatosis: an analysis of 158 patients. Ann Intern Med 1992;116:488-98.
9. Hoffman GS, Leavitt RY, Fleisher TA, Minor JR, Fauci AS. Treatment of Wegener's granulomatosis with intermittent high-dose intravenous cyclophosphamide. Am J Med 1990;89:403-10.
10. Langford CA, Sneller MC. Biologic therapies in the vasculitides. Current Opinion in Rheumatol 2003;15:3-10.
11. Hoffman GS, Thomas-Golbanov CK, Chan J, Akst LM, Eliachar I. Treatment of subglottic stenosis due to Wegener's granulomatosis with intralesional corticosteroids and dilation. J Rheumatol 2003;30:1017-21.

CHAPTER 16 – RELAPSING POLYCHONDRITIS

1. Kent PD, Michet CJ Jr, Luthra HS. Relapsing polychondritis. Current Opinion in Rheumatology. 2004;16:56-61.
2. Balsa A, Expinosa A, Cuesta M, et al. Joint symptoms in relapsing polychondritis. Clin Exp Rheumatol 1995;13:425-30.
3. Bowness P, Hawley IC, Dearden A, Walport MJ. Complete heart block and severe aortic incompetence in relapsing polychondritis; clinicopathologic findings. Arthritis Rheum 34:97–100, 1991.
4. Trentham DE, Le CH. Relapsing polychondritis. Ann Intern Med 1998;129:114-22.
5. Michet CJ, Jr., McKenna CH, Luthra HS, O'Fallon WM. Relapsing polychondritis. Survival and predictive role of early disease manifestations. Ann Intern Med 1986;104:74-8.

CHAPTER 17 – BEHÇET'S SYNDROME

1. Anonymous. Criteria for diagnosis of Behçet's disease. International Study Group for Behçet's Disease. Lancet 1990;335(8697):1078-80.
2. Mutlu S, Scully C. The person behind the eponym: Hulusi Behçet (1889-1948). Journal of Oral Pathology & Medicine 1994;23:289-90.
3. Sakane T, Takeno M, Suzuki N, Inaba G. Behçet's disease. N Engl J Med 1999;341:1284-91.
4. Yazici H, Yurdakul S, Hamuryudan V. Behçet disease. Current Opinion in Rheumatology 2001;13:18-22.

5. Saeny A, Ausejo M, Shea B, et al. Pharmacotherapy of Behçet's syndrome. Cochrane Database of Systematic Reviews 2000;CD001084.

CHAPTER 18 – THE (SERONEGATIVE) SPONDYLOARTHRITIDES

1. Gladman DD. Clinical aspects of the spondyloarthropathies. Am J Med Sci 1998;316:234-8.
2. Reveille JD. HLA-B27 and the seronegative spondyloarthropathies. Am J Med Sci 1998;316:239-49.
3. Baech J, Schmidt-Olsen S, Steffensen R,Varming K, Grunnet N, Jersild C. Frequency of HLA-B27 subtypes in a Danish population and in Danish patients with ankylosing spondylitis. Tissue Antigens 1997;49:499-502.
4. Brown MA, Jepson A, Young A, Whittle HC, Greenwood BM, Wordsworth BP. Ankylosing spondylitis in West Africans--evidence for a non-HLA-B27 protective effect. Ann Rheum Dis 1997;56:68-70.
5. Gladman, DD. Clinical manifestations and diagnosis of psoriatic arthritis. In: UpToDate, Rose, BD (Ed), UpToDate, Wellesley, MA, 2004.
6. Earwaker JW, Cotten A. SAPHO: syndrome or concept? Imaging findings. Skeletal Radiol 2003;32:311-27.
7. Santos H, Brophy S, Calin A. Exercise in ankylosing spondylitis: how much is optimum? J Rheumatol 1998;25:2156-60.
8. Clegg DO, Reda DJ, Abdellatif M. Comparison of sulfasalazine and placebo for the treatment of axial and peripheral articular manifestations of the seronegative spondylarthropathies: a Department of Veterans Affairs cooperative study Arthritis & Rheumatism 1999;42:2325-9.
9. Jones G, Crotty M, Brooks P. Interventions for psoriatic arthritis. Cochrane Database of Systematic Reviews 2000:CD000212.
10. Leirisalo-Repo M. Therapeutic aspects of spondyloarthropathies -- a review. Scand J Rheumatol 1998;27:323-8.

CHAPTER 19 – SARCOID ARTHRITIS

1. O'Gradaigh D, Hazelman B: Miscellaneous conditions presenting to the rheumatologist. In: Oxford textbook of Medicine, 4th edition. Warrell DA, Cox TM, Firth JD (eds.): Oxford University Press. 2003 3.120-7.
2. Baughman RP. Pulmonary sarcoidosis. Clinics in Chest Medicine 2004;25:521-30.
3. Zisman DA, Shorr, AF, Lynch JP: Sarcoidosis involving the musculoskeletal system. Semin Resp Crit Care Med 23:555–570, 2002.
4. Pettersson T. Sarcoid and erythema nodosum arthropathies. Best Practice & Research in Clinical Rheumatology. 2000;14:461-76.
5. Visser H, Vos K, Zanelli E, et al: Sarcoid arthritis: clinical characteristics, diagnostic aspects, and risk factors. Ann Rheum Dis 61:499–504, 2002.

CHAPTER 20 – CRYSTAL INDUCED ARTHRITIS, GOUT AND PSEUDOGOUT

1. Schumacher HR. Crystal-induced arthritis: an overview. Am J Med 1996;100:46S-52S.
2. Sack K. Monarthritis: differential diagnosis. Am J Med 1997;102(1A):30S-34S.
3. Wortmann RL: Gout and other disorders of purine metabolism. In: Fauci AS, Braunwald E, Isselbacher KJ, Wilson JD, Martin JB, Casper DL, Hauser SL, Longo DL eds. Harrison's Principles of Internal Medicine, 14th ed. New York: McGraw-Hill 1998; 2158-66.
4. Emmerson BT. The management of gout. N Engl J Med 1996;334:445-51.
5. Sandor V, Hassan R, Kohn E. Exacerbation of pseudogout by granulocyte colony-stimulating factor [letter]. Ann Intern Med 1996;125:781.
6. Ryan LM: Calcium pyrophosphate dihydrate crystal deposition. In: Klippel J, Weyand CM, Wortmann RL eds. Primer on the Rheumatic Diseases, 11th ed. Atlanta GA: The Arthritis Foundation 1997; 226-9.

CHAPTER 21 – SEPTIC (BACTERIAL) ARTHRITIS

1. Goldenberg DL. Septic arthritis. Lancet 1998;351(9097):197-202.
2. Juárez M, Misischia R, Alarcón GS. Infections in systemic connective tissue diseases: systemic lupus erythematosus, scleroderma, and polymyositis/dermatomyositis. Rheumatic Disease Clinics of North America 2003:29;163-84.
3. Gupta MN, Sturrock RD, Field M A Prospective 2-year study of 75 patients with adult-onset septic arthritis. Rheumatology 2001; 40:24-30
4. Kaandorp CJE, Dinaut HJ, VanderLaar MAFP, et el. Incidence and sources of native and prosthetic joint infection: a community-based prospective study. Annals of Rheumatic Diseases 1997;56:470-475.
5. Louie JS, Liebling MR. The polymerase chain reaction in infectious and post-infectious arthritis: a review. Rheumatic Disease Clinics of North America 1998;24:227-36.
6. Garcia-De La Torre, I. Advances in the Management of Septic Arthritis. Rheumatic Disease Clinics of North America 2003;29:61-75.
7. Sack K. Monarthritis: differential diagnosis. Am J Med 1997;102 (1A):30S-34S.
8. O'Brien JP, Goldenberg DL, Rice PA. Disseminated gonococcal infection: a prospective analysis of 49 patients and a review of pathophysiology and immune mechanisms. Medicine (Baltimore) 1983;62:395-406.

CHAPTER 22 – OTHER INFECTIOUS ARTHRITIDES

LYME DISEASE

1. Steere AC, Malawista SE, Snydman DR, et al. Lyme arthritis: an epidemic of oligoarticular arthritis in children and adults in three Connecticut communities. Arthritis & Rheumatism 1977;20:7-17.

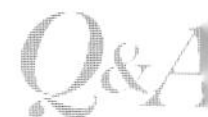

2. Steere AC. Lyme disease. New England Journal of Medicine 2001;345:115-125.
3. Sigal LH. Toward a more complete appreciation of the clinical spectrum of Borrelia burgdorferi infection: early Lyme disease without erythema migrans. American Journal of Medicine [editorial] 2003;114:74-5.
4. Nadelman RB, Wormser GP. Lyme borreliosis. Lancet 1998;352:557-65.
5. Klempner MS, Schmid CH, Hu L, et al. Intralaboratory reliability of serologic and urine testing for Lyme disease. American Journal of Medicine 2001;110:217-9.
6. Wormser GP, Nadelman RB, Dattwyler RJ, et al. Practice guidelines for the treatment of Lyme disease. Clin Infect Dis 2000; 31(Suppl 1):S1-14.
7. Wormser GP, Ramanathan R, Nowakowski J, et al. Duration of antibiotic therapy for early Lyme disease. A randomized, double-blind, placebo-controlled trial. Ann Intern Med 2003;138:697-04.
8. Karlsson M, Hammers-Berggren S, Lindquist L, et.al. Comparison of intravenous penicillin G and oral doxycycline for treatment of Lyme neuroborreliosis. Neurology 1994;44:1203-7.
9. Shadick NA, Liang MH, Phillips CB. The cost-effectiveness of vaccination against Lyme disease. Archives of Internal Medicine 2001;161:554-61.
10. Thanassi WT, Schoen RT. The Lyme disease vaccine: Conception, development, and implementation. Ann Intern Med 2000;132:661-8.

VIRAL ARTHRITIDES

1. Ytterberg SR. Viral arthritis. Current Opinion in Rheumatology. 1999;11:275-80.
2. Young NS, Brown KE. Parvovirus B19. N Engl J Med 2004;350:586-97.
3. Cuellar ML, Espinoza LR. Rheumatic manifestations of HIV-AIDS. Best Practice & Research in Clinical Rheumatology 2000;14:579-93.
4. Ganem D, Prince AM. Hepatitis B virus infection--natural history and clinical consequences. N Engl J Med 2004;350:1118-29.
5. Olivieri I, Palazzi C, Padula A. Hepatitis C virus and arthritis. Rheumatic Diseases Clinics of North America 2003;29:111-22.
6. Kalish RA, Knopf AN, Gary GW, Canoso JJ. Lupus-like presentation of human parvovirus B19 infection. J Rheuamtol 1992;19:169-71.
7. Scroggie DA, Carpenter MT, Cooper RI, Higgs JB. Parvovirus arthropathy outbreak in southwestern United States. J Rheumatol 2000;27:2444-8.
8. Naides SJ, Scharosch LL, Foto F, Howard EJ. Rheumatologic manifestations of human parvovirus B19 infection in adults. Initial two-year clinical experience. Arthritis & Rheumatism 1990;33:1297-309.
9. Gran JT, Johnsen V, Myklebust G, Nordbo SA. The variable clinical picture of arthritis induced by human parvovirus B19. Report of seven adult cases and review of the literature. Scandinavian Journal of Rheumatology 1995; 24:174-9.
10. Frickhofen N, Abkowitz, JL, Saffoid M, et al. Persistent B19 parvovirus infection in patients infected with human immunodeficiency virus type 1 (HIV-1): A treatable cause of anemia in AIDS. Ann Intern Med 1990;113:926-33.
11. Jobanputra P, Davidson F, Graham S, et al. High frequency of parvovirus B19 in patients tested for rheumatoid factor. BMJ 1995;311(7019):1542.

12. Soloninka CA, Anderson MJ, Laskin CA, Anti-DNA and antilymphocyte antibodies during acute infection with human parvovirus B19. J Rheumatol 1989;16:777-81.

TUBERCULOUS ARTHRITIS

1. Ytterberg SR: Infectious disorders. D. Mycobacterial, fungal, and parasitic arthritis. In: Klippel JH (ed): Primer on the Rheumatic Diseases, 12th ed., 2001. Atlanta, The Arthritis Foundation, p 274-279.
2. Sembekar A, Babhulkar S. Chemotherapy for osteoarticular tuberculosis. Clin Orthop 2002;398:20.

CHAPTER 23 – RS3PE SYNDROME

1. McCarty DJ, O'Duffy JD, Pearson L, Hunter JB. Remitting seronegative symmetrical synovitis with pitting edema. RS3PE syndrome. JAMA 1985;254:2763-7.
2. Schaeverbeke T, Fatour E, Marce S, et. al. Remitting seronegative symmetric synovitis with pitting oedema: disease or syndrome? Ann Rheum Dis 1995;54:681-4.
3. Olivieri I, Salvarani C, Cantini F. RS3PE syndrome: an overview. Clin Exp Rheumatol 2000;18(4 Suppl 20):S53-5.

CHAPTER 24 – FIBRODYSPLASIA (MYOSITIS) OSSIFICANS PROGRESSIVA

1. Bridges AJ, Hsu KC, Singh A, Churchill R, Miles J. Fibrodysplasia (myositis) ossificans progressiva. Seminars in Arthritis & Rheumatism 1994;24:155-64.
2. Siegert JJ, Wortmann RL. Myositis ossificans simulating acute monoarticular arthritis. J Rheumatol 1986;13:652-4.
3. Connor JM, Evans DA. Fibrodysplasia ossificans progressiva. The clinical features and natural history of 34 patients. Journal of Bone & Joint Surgery - British Volume 1982;64:76-83.
4. Russell RG, Smith R, Bishop MC, Price DA. Treatment of myositis ossificans progressiva with a diphosphonate. Lancet 1972;1(7740):10-1.

CHAPTER 25 – REFLEX SYMPATHETIC DYSTROPHY

1. Turner-Stokes L. Reflex sympathetic dystrophy--a complex regional pain syndrome. Disability & Rehabilitation 2002;24:939-47.
2. Raja SN, Grabow TS. Complex regional pain syndrome I (reflex sympathetic dystrophy). Anesthesiology 2002;96:1254-60.
3. Baron R, Schattschmeider J, Binder A, et al. Relation between sympathetic vasomotor activity and pain and hyperalgesia in complex regional pain syndromes. A case-control study. Lancet 2002;359:1655-60.

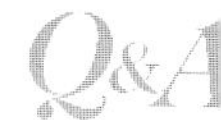

4. van de Beek WJ, Schwartzman RJ, van Nes SI, et al. Diagnostic criteria used in studies of reflex sympathetic dystrophy. Neurology 2002;58:522-6.
5. Steinbrocker O, Argyros TG. The shoulder-hand syndrome: present status as a diagnostic and therapeutic entity. Med Clin North AM 1958;42:1533-1553.
6. Todorovic-Tirnanic m, Obradovic V, Han R, et al. Diagnostic approach to reflex sympathetic dystrophy after fracture: radiography or bone scintigraphy? Eur J Nucl Med 1995:22:1187-93.
7. Ushida T, Tani T, Kanbara T, et al. Analgesic effects of ketamine ointment in patients with complex regional pain syndrome type I. Regional Anesthesia and Pain Medicine 2002;27:524-8.
8. Kemler MA, Barendse GA, van Kleef M, et al. Spinal cord stimulation in patients with chronic reflex sympathetic dystrophy. N Engl J Med 2000;343:618-24.

CHAPTER 26 – CARPAL TUNNEL SYNDROME

1. Biundo JJ: Musculoskeletal signs and symptoms. D. Regional rheumatic pain syndromes. In: Klippel JH (ed): Primer on the Rheumatic Diseases, 12th ed., 2001. Atlanta, The Arthritis Foundation, p 174-188.
2. Stevens JC, Beard CM, O'Fallon WM, Kurland LT. Conditions associated with carpal tunnel syndrome. Mayo Clin Proc 1992;67:541-8.

CHAPTER 27 – POPLITEAL (BAKER'S) CYST

1. Biundo JJ: Regional rheumatic pain syndromes. In: Klippel J, Weyand CM, Wortmann RL eds. Primer on the Rheumatic Diseases, 11th ed. Atlanta GA: The Arthritis Foundation 1997; 136-48.
2 Drescher MJ, Smally AJ. Thrombophlebitis and pseudothrombophlebitis in the ED. Am J Emerg Med 1997;15:683-5.

CHAPTER 28 – OTHER BURSITIDES AND TENDINITIDES

1. Sheon RP, Moskowitz RW, Goldberg, VM. Soft Tissue Rheumatic Pain: Recognition, Management, Prevention, 3d ed, Williams Wilkins, Baltimore, 1996.
2. Zimmermann B 3rd, Mikolich DJ, Ho G Jr. Septic bursitis. Semin Arthritis Rheum 1995;24:391-410.

CHAPTER 29 – SELECTED DERMATO-ARTHRITIDES

ERYTHEMA NODOSUM

1. Mert A, Ozaras R, Tabak F, et al. Erythema nodosum: an experience of 10 years. Scandinavian Journal of Infectious Diseases 2004;36:424-7.
2. Garcia-Porrua C, Gonzalez-Gay MA, Vazquez-Caruncho M, et al. Erythema nodosum: etiologic and predictive factors in a defined population. Arthritis Rheum 2000;43:584-92.

SWEET'S SYNDROME

1. von den Driesch P. Sweet's syndrome (acute febrile neutrophilic dermatosis). J Am Acad Dermatol 1994;31:535-56.
2. Kemmett D, Hunter JA. Sweet's syndrome: a clinicopathologic review of twenty-nine cases. J Am Acad Dermatol 1990;23(Pt 1)503-7.

CHAPTER 30 – THERAPEUTICS

1. Fries JF. The epidemiology of NSAID gastropathy: the ARAMIS experience. J Clin Rheumatol 1998;4:S11.
2. Wolfe MM, Lichtenstein DR, Singh G: Gastrointestinal toxicity of nonsteroidal antiinflammatory drugs. New Engl J Med 1999;341:1397-9.
3. Bresalier RS, Sandler RS, Quan H, et al. Cardiovascular events associated with rofecoxib in a colorectal adenoma chemoprevention trial. N Engl J Med 2005;352:1092-1102.
4. Bombardier C, Laine L, Reicin A, et al. Comparison of upper gastrointestinal toxicity of rofecoxib and naproxen in patients with rheumatoid arthritis. VIGOR Study Group. N Engl J Med 2000;343:1520-8, 2 p following 1528.
5. Fitzgerald GA. Coxibs and cardiovascular disease. N Engl J Med 2004;351:1709-11.
6. Finckh A, Aronson MD. Cardiovascular risks of cyclooxygenase-2 inhibitors: Where we stand now. (Editorial) Ann Int Med 2005; 142:212-214.
7. Kimmel SE, Berlin JA, Reilly M, Jaskowiak J, Kishel L, Chittams J, Strom BL. The effects of nonselective non-aspirin non-steroidal anti-inflammatory medications on the risk of nonfatal myocardial infarction and their interaction with aspirin. Journal of the American College of Cardiology 2004;43:985-90.
8. Gubner R, August TS, Ginsberg V. Therapeutic suppression of tissue reactivity. II. Effect of aminopterin in rheumatoid arthritis and psoriasis. Am J Med Sci 1951; 221:176-82.
9. Maravic M, Bologna C, Daures JP, et al. Radiologic progression in early rheumatoid arthritis treated with methotrexate. J Rheumatol 1999;26:262-7.
10. Kremer JM. Safety, efficacy, and mortality in a long-term cohort of patients with rheumatoid arthritis taking methotrexate: followup after a mean of 13.3 years. Arthritis Rheum 1997;40:984-5.
11. Cronstein BN, Naime D, Ostad E. The antiinflammatory mechanism of methotrexate: increased adenosine release at inflamed sites diminishes leukocyte accumulation in an in vivo model of inflammation. J Clin Invest 1993;92:2675-82.
12. Barrera P, Boerbooms AMT, Janssen EM, et al: Circulating soluble tumor necrosis factor receptors, interleukin-2 receptors, tumor necrosis factor-α, and interleukin-6 levels in rheumatoid arthritis: longitudinal evaluation during methotrexate and azathioprine therapy. Arthritis Rheum 1993;36:1070-9.
13. O'Dell, Leff R, Paulsen G, et al. Treatment of rheumatoid arthritis with methotrexate and hydroxychloroquine, methotrexate and sulfasalazine, or a combination of the three medications: results of a two-year, randomized, double-blind, placebo-controlled trial. Arthritis Rheum 2002;46:1164-70
14. Choi HK, Hernan MA, Seeger JD, et al. Methotrexate and mortality in patients with rheumatoid arthritis: a prospective study. Lancet 2002;359(9313):1173-7.

15. Fox, R. Antimalarial drugs. In: Koopman WJ, ed. Arthritis and Allied Conditions, A Textbook of Rheumatology, 13th ed. Baltimore:Williams and Wilkins 1997; 671-78.
16. Day RO. SAARDs. In: Klippel JH, Dieppe PA eds. Rheumatology, 2nd ed. London: Mosby 1998;3.8.1-3.8.10.
17. In: Physicians' Desk Reference. Montvale NJ: Medical Economics Company, Inc 2000.
18. In: McEvoy GK ed. AHFS (American Hospital Formulary Service) Drug Information. Bethesda: The American Society of Health-System Pharmacists, Inc 2000. 188
19. Hamilton E, Scott J. Hydroxychloroquine in treatment of rheumatoid arthritis. Arthritis & Rheumatism 1962;5:502-12.
20. Anonymous. A randomized study of the effect of withdrawing hydroxychloroquine sulfate in systemic lupus erythematosus. The Canadian Hydroxychloroquine Study Group. N Engl J Med 1991;324:150-4.
21. Fox, RI: Sjogren's syndrome. In: Klippel J, Weyand CM, Wortmann RL eds. Primer on the Rheumatic Diseases, 11th ed. Atlanta,GA: The Arthritis Foundation 1997; 283-88.
22. Bernstein HN. Ocular safety of hydroxychloroquine. Annals of Ophthalmology 1991;23:292.
23. Svartz N. Salazopyrin, a new sulfanilamide preparation. Acta Med Scand 1942;110:577.
24. Amos RS. The history of the use of sulphasalazine in rheumatology. Br J Rheumatol 1995;34 Suppl 2:2-6.
25. McConkey B, Amos RS, Durham S, et al. Sulphasalazine in rheumatoid arthritis. Br Med J 1980;16;280(6212):442-4.
26. Box SA, Pullar T. Sulphasalazine in the treatment of rheumatoid arthritis. Br J Rheumatol 1997;36:382-6.
27. O'Dell JR, Leff R, Paulsen G, et al. Treatment of rheumatoid arthritis with methotrexate and hydroxychloroquine, methotrexate and sulfasalazine, or a combination of the three medications: results of a two-year, randomized, double-blind, placebo-controlled trial. Arthritis Rheum 2002;46:1164-70.
28. American College of Rheumatology Ad Hoc Committee on Clinical Guidelines: Guidelines for monitoring drug therapy in rheumatoid arthritis. Arthritis Rheum 1996;39:723-31.
29. Ferraz MB, Tugwell P, Goldsmith CH, et al: Meta-analysis of sulfasalazine in ankylosing spondylitis. J Rheumatol 1990;17:1482-6.
30. Clegg DO, Reda DJ, Mejias E, et al: Comparison of sulfasalazine and placebo in the treatment of psoriatic arthritis. Arthritis Rheum 1996;39:2013-20.
31. Weinblatt ME, Reda D, Henderson W, et al. Sulfasalazine treatment for rheumatoid arthritis: a metaanalysis of 15 randomized trials. J Rheumatol 1999;26:2123-30.
32. van Riel PL, van Gestel AM, van de Putte LB. Long-term usage and side effect profile of sulphasalazine in rheumatoid arthritis. Br J Rheumatol 1995;34 Suppl 2:40-2.
33. Yu LP Jr, Smith GN Jr, Hasty KA, Brandt KD. Doxycycline inhibits type XI collagenolytic activity of extracts from human osteoarthritic cartilage and of gelatinase. J Rheumatol 1991;18:1450-2.
34. Kloppenburg M, Breedveld FC, Terwiel JP, Mallee C, Dijkmans BA. Minocycline in active rheumatoid arthritis. A double-blind, placebo-controlled trial. Arthritis Rheum 1994;37:629-36.
35. Tilley BC, Alarcon GS, Heyse SP, et al. Minocycline in rheumatoid arthritis: A 48-week, double-blind, placebo-controlled trial. Ann Int Med 1995;122:81–89.
36. O'Dell JR, Paulsen G, Haire CE, et al. Treatment of early seropositive rheumatoid arthritis with minocycline: four-year followup of a double-blind, placebo-controlled trial. Arthritis Rheum 1999;42:1691-5.

37. Fox RI. Mechanism of action of leflunomide in rheumatoid arthritis. J Rheumatol Suppl 1998;53:20-6.

38. Hoi, A, Littlejohn, GO. Aminotransferase levels during treatment of rheumatoid arthritis with leflunomide in clinical practice. Ann Rheum Dis 2003;62:379-379.

39. In: Kastrup EK ed. Drug Facts and Comparisons. St. Louis MO:Wolters Kluwer 1999.

40. Mladenovic V, Domljan Z, Rozman B, et al. Safety and effectiveness of leflunomide in the treatment of patients with active rheumatoid arthritis. Arthritis Rheum 1995;38:1595-603.

41. Sharp JT, Strand V, Leung H, et al. Treatment with leflunomide slows radiographic progression of rheumatoid arthritis: results from three randomized controlled trials of leflunomide in patients with active rheumatoid arthritis. Leflunomide Rheumatoid Arthritis Investigators Group. Arthritis Rheum 2000;43:495-505.

42. Strand V, Cohen S, Schiff M, et al. Treatment of active rheumatoid arthritis with leflunomide compared with placebo and methotrexate. Leflunomide Rheumatoid Arthritis Investigators Group. Arch Intern Med 1999;159:2542-2550.

43. Emery P, Breedveld FC, Lemmel EM, et al. A comparison of the efficacy and safety of leflunomide and methotrexate for the treatment of rheumatoid arthritis. Rheumatology (Oxford) 2000;39:655-65.

44. In: McEvoy GK ed.AHFS (American Hospital Formulary Service) Drug Information. Bethesda: The American Society of Health-System Pharmacists, Inc 2000.)

45. O'Dell JR, Leff R, Paulsen G, et al. Treatment of rheumatoid arthritis with methotrexate and hydroxychloroquine, methotrexate and sulfasalazine, or a combination of the three medications: results of a two-year, randomized, double-blind, placebo-controlled trial. Arthritis Rheum 2002;46:1164-70.

46. Haagsma CJ, van Riel PL, de Rooij DJ, Vree TB, et al. Combination of methotrexate and sulphasalazine vs methotrexate alone: a randomized open clinical trial in rheumatoid arthritis patients resistant to sulphasalazine therapy. Br J Rheumatol 1994;33:1049-55.

47. Boers M, Verhoeven AC, Markusse HM, et al. Randomised comparison of combined step-down prednisolone, methotrexate and sulphasalazine with sulphasalazine alone in early rheumatoid arthritis. Lancet 1997;350(9074):309-18.

48. Mottonen T, Hannonen P, Leirisalo-Repo M, et al. Comparison of combination therapy with single-drug therapy in early rheumatoid arthritis: a randomised trial. FIN-RACo trial group. Lancet 1999;353(9164):1568-73.

49. Weinblatt ME, Kremer JM, Coblyn JS, et al. Pharmacokinetics, safety, and efficacy of combination treatment with methotrexate and leflunomide in patients with active rheumatoid arthritis. Arthritis Rheum 1999;42:1322-8.

50. Kremer JM, Genovese MC, Cannon GW, et al. Concomitant leflunomide therapy in patients with active rheumatoid arthritis despite stable doses of methotrexate. A randomized, double-blind, placebo-controlled trial. Ann Intern Med 2002;137:726-3.

51. Weinblatt ME, Kremer JM, Bankhurst AD, et al. A trial of etanercept, a recombinant tumor necrosis factor receptor:Fc fusion protein, in patients with rheumatoid arthritis receiving methotrexate. N Engl J Med 1999;340:253-9.

52. Maini RN, Breedveld FC, Kalden JR, et al. Sustained improvement over two years in physical function, structural damage, and signs and symptoms among patients with rheumatoid arthritis treated with infliximab and methotrexate. Arthritis Rheum 2004;50:1051-65.

53. Keystone EC, Kavanaugh AF, Sharp JT, et al. Radiographic, clinical, and functional outcomes of treatment with adalimumab (a human anti-tumor necrosis factor monoclonal antibody) in patients with active rheumatoid arthritis receiving concomitant methotrexate therapy: a randomized, placebo-controlled, 52-week trial. Arthritis Rheum 2004;50:1400-11.

54. Landewe RB, Boers M, Verhoeven AC, et al. COBRA combination therapy in patients with early rheumatoid arthritis: long-term structural benefits of a brief intervention. Arthritis Rheum 46:347-56, 2002.

55. Schiff M. Emerging treatments for rheumatoid arthritis. Am J Med 1997;102(1A):11S-15S.

56. Conaghan PG, Lehmann T, Brooks P. Disease-modifying antirheumatic drugs. Curr Opin Rheumatol 1997;9:183-90.

57. Moreland LW, Heck LW, Jr., Koopman WJ. Biologic agents for treating rheumatoid arthritis. Concepts and progress. Arthritis & Rheumatism 1997;40:397-409.

58. Moreland LW, Schiff MH, Baumgartner SW, et al. Etanercept therapy in rheumatoid arthritis. A randomized, controlled trial. Ann Intern Med 1999;130:478-86.

59. Mease PJ, Goffe BS, Metz J, VanderStoep A, Finck B, Burge DJ. Etanercept in the treatment of psoriatic arthritis and psoriasis: a randomized trial. Lancet. 2000;356(9227):385-90.

60. Davis JC Jr, Van Der Heijde D, Braun J. Enbrel Ankylosing Spondylitis Study Group. Recombinant human tumor necrosis factor receptor (etanercept) for treating ankylosing spondylitis: a randomized controlled trial. Arthritis Rheum. 2003;48:3230-6.

61. Genovese MC, Bathon JM, Martin RW, et al. Etanercept versus methotrexate in early rheumatoid arthritis: two year radiographic and clinical outcomes. Arthritis Rheum. 2002;46:1443-50.

62. In: Kastrup EK ed.Drug Facts and Comparisons. St. Louis MO:Wolters Kluwer 1999.

63. Brown, SL, Greene MH, Gershon SK, Edwards ET, Braun MM. Tumor necrosis factor antagonist therapy and lymphoma development: twenty six cases reported to the Food and Drug Administration. Arthritis Rheum. 2002;46:3151-8.

64. Weinblatt ME, Kremer JM, Bankhurst AD, et al. A trial of etanercept, a recombinant tumor necrosis factor receptor:Fc fusion protein, in patients with rheumatoid arthritis receiving methotrexate. N Engl J Med 1999;340:253-9.

65. Goldenberg MM. Etanercept, a novel drug for the treatment of patients with severe, active rheumatoid arthritis. Clin Ther 1999;21:75-87 (discussion 1-2).

66. Orozco C, Dao K, Cush JJ, et al. Safety of TNF inhibitors during pregnancy in patients with inflammatory arthritis. Arthritis & Rheum 2005;

67. Carter JD, Valeriano J, Vasey FB. Tumor necrosis factor alpha inhibition and VATER association: a causal relationship? J Rheum (in press).

68. Maini R, St. Clair EW, Breedveld F, et al. Infliximab (chimeric anti-tumor necrosis factor alpha monoclonal antibody) versus placebo in rheumatoid arthritis patients receiving concomitant methotrexate: a randomised phase III trial. ATTRACT Study Group. Lancet. 1999;354(9194):1932-9.

69. Ruderman EM, Markenson JA. Granulomatous infections and tumor necrosis factor antagonist therapy: update through June 2002 (abstract). Arthritis Rheum 2003;48:S241.

70. Gardam MA, Keystone EC, Menzies R, et al. Anti-tumor necrosis factor agents and tuberculosis risk: mechanisms of action and clinical management. Lancet Infect Dis. 2003;3(3):148-55.

71. Brown SL, Greene MH, Gershon SK, et al. Tumor necrosis factor antagonist therapy and lymphoma development: twenty six cases reported to the Food and Drug Administration. Arthritis Rheum. 2002;46:3151-8.

72. Weinblatt ME, Keystone EC, Furst DE, et al. Adalimumab, a fully human anti-tumor necrosis factor alpha monoclonal antibody, for the treatment of rheumatoid arthritis in patients taking concomitant methotrexate: the ARMADA trial. Arthritis Rheum 2003;48:35-45.

73. Den Broeder AA, Joosten LA, Saxne T, et al. Long term anti-tumor necrosis factor alpha monotherapy in rheumatoid arthritis: effect on radiological course and prognostic value of markers of cartilage turnover and endothelial activation. Ann Rheum Dis. 2002;61:311-8.

74. Wollheim FA. TNF inhibition as a therapy for rheumatoid arthritis. Expert Opin Invest Drugs. 2002;11:947-53.

75. Furst DE, Schiff MH, Fleischmann RM, et al. Adalimumab, a fully human anti tumor necrosis factor-alpha monoclonal antibody, and concomitant standard antirheumatic therapy for the treatment of rheumatoid arthritis: results of STAR (Safety Trial of Adalimumab in Rheumatoid Arthritis). J Rheumatol 2003;30:2563-71.

76. O'Dell JR. Drug therapy: Therapeutic strategies for rheumatoid arthritis. N Eng J Med 2004;350:2591-602.

77. Olsen NJ, Stein CM. Drug therapy: New drugs for rheumatoid arthritis. N Eng J Med 2004;350:2167-79.

78. Jiang Y, Genant HK, Watt I, et al. A multicenter, double-blind, dose-ranging, randomized, placebo-controlled study of recombinant human interleukin-1 receptor antagonist in patients with rheumatoid arthritis: radiologic progression and correlation of Genant and Larsen scores. Arthritis Rheum 2000;43:1001-9.

79. Shergy WJ, Cohen S, Greenwald M, et al: Anakinra inhibits the progression of radiographically measured joint destruction in rheumatoid arthritis. Arthritis Rheum 2002;46:3420.

80. Cohen S, Hurd E, Cush J, et al. Treatment of rheumatoid arthritis with anakinra, a recombinant human interleukin-1 receptor antagonist, in combination with methotrexate: results of a twenty-four-week, multicenter, randomized, double-blind, placebo-controlled trial. Arthritis Rheum 2002;46:614-24.

81. Weisman MH. What are the risks of biologic therapy in rheumatoid arthritis? An update on safety. J Rheumatol Suppl 2002;65:33-8.

82. Wiesenhutter CW, Irish BL, Bertram JR. Treatment of patients with refractory rheumatoid arthritis with extracorporeal protein A immunoadsorption columns: A pilot trial. J Rheumatol 1994;21:804-12.

83. Felson DT, LaValley MP, Baldassare AR, Block JA, Caldwell JR, Cannon GW, et al. The Prosorba column for treatment of refractory rheumatoid arthritis: a randomized, double-blind, sham-controlled trial. Arthritis Rheum 1999;42:2153-9.

84. In: McEvoy GK ed. AHFS (American Hospital Formulary Service) Drug Information. Bethesda: The American Society of Health-System Pharmacists, Inc 2000.

85. Rubin CT, Rubin JE: The biology, physiology, and morphology of bone. In: Kelley WN, Harris ED, Ruddy S, Sledge CB eds. Textbook of Rheumatology, 5th ed. Philadelphia PA: W.B. Saunders Company 1997; 55-75.

86. In: Physicians' Desk Reference. Montvale NJ: Medical Economics Company, Inc 2000.

87. Siris ES: Paget's disease of bone. In: Favus MJ, ed. Primer on the Metabolic Bone Diseases and Disorders of Mineral Metabolism, 4th ed. Philadelphia PA: Lippincott, Williams and Wilkins 1999; 415-25.

88. Kapetanos G, Symeonides PP, Dimitriou C, et al. A double blind study of intranasal calcitonin for established postmenopausal osteoporosis. Acta Orthop Scand Suppl 1997;275:108-11.

89. Overgaard K, Hansen MA, Jensen SB, Christiansen C. Effect of salcatonin given intranasally on bone mass and fracture rates in established osteoporosis: a dose-response study. Br Med J 1992;305(6853):556-61.

90. Waldburger M, Meier JL, Gobelet C. The frozen shoulder: diagnosis and treatment. Prospective study of 50 cases of adhesive capsulitis. Clin Rheumatol 1992;11:364-8.

91. Ritchlin CT: Reflex sympathetic dystrophy and transient regional osteoporosis. In: Klippel J,Weyand CM,Wortmann RL eds. Primer on the Rheumatic Diseases, 11th ed. Atlanta GA: The Arthritis Foundation 1997; 319-21.

92. Paice E. Reflex sympathetic dystrophy. Br Med J 1995;310(6995):1645-8.

93. Maksymowych WP. Managing acute osteoporotic vertebral fractures with calcitonin. Can Fam Physician 1998;44:2160-6.

94. Silverman SL. Nasal calcitonin. Endocrine 1997;6:199-202.

95. Andrews WC. What's new in preventing and treating osteoporosis? Postgrad Med 1998;104:89-92, 95-7.

96. Dempster DW, Cosman F, Parisien M, et al. Anabolic actions of parathyroid hormone on bone. Endocr Rev 1993;14:690-709.

97. Jiang Y, Zhao JJ, Mitlak BH, et al. Recombinant human parathyroid hormone (1-34) [teriparatide] improves both cortical and cancellous bone structure. J Bone Miner Res 2003;18:1932-41.

98. Crandall C. Parathyroid hormone for treatment of osteoporosis. Arch Intern Med 2002;11;162:2297-309.

99. Rittmaster RS, Bolognese M, Ettinger MP. Enhancement of bone mass in osteoporotic women with parathyroid hormone followed by alendronate. J Clin Endocrinol Metab 2000;85:2129–34.

100. Black DM, Greenspan SL, Ensrud KE, et al. PaTH Study Investigators. The effects of parathyroid hormone and alendronate alone or in combination in postmenopausal osteoporosis. N Engl J Medicine 2003;349:1207-15.

101. Pak CY, Sakhaee K, Adams-Huet B, et al. Treatment of postmenopausal osteoporosis with slow-release sodium fluoride. Final report of a randomized controlled trial. Ann Intern Med 1995;123:401-8.

102. Reginster JY, Meurmans L, Zegels B, et al. The effect of sodium monofluorophosphate plus calcium on vertebral fracture rate in postmenopausal women with moderate osteoporosis. A randomized, controlled trial. Ann Intern Med 1998;129:1-8.

103. American College Of Rheumatology Ad Hoc Committee On Glucocorticoid-Induced Osteoporosis. Recommendations for the prevention and treatment of glucocorticoid-induced osteoporosis. 2001 update. Arthritis Rheum 2001;44:1496-1503.

104. Schmacher HR, Chen, LX. Injectable corticosteroids in treatment of arthritis of the knee. Am J Med 2005;118:1208-1214.

105. Schnitzer TJ, Burmester GR, Mysler E, et al. Comparison of lumiracoxib with naproxen and ibuprofen in the Therapeutic Arthritis Research and Gastrointestinal Event Trial (TARGET), reduction in ulcer complications: randomised controlled trial. Lancet. 2004;364:665-74.

106. Farkouh ME, Kirshner H, Harrington RA, et al. Comparison of lumiracoxib with naproxen and ibuprofen in the Therapeutic Arthritis Research and Gastrointestinal Event Trial (TARGET), cardiovascular outcomes: randomised controlled trial. Lancet. 2004;364:675-84.

107. Hart L. Lumiracoxib reduced ulcer complications compared with ibuprofen and naproxen in OA and did not increase cardiovascular outcomes. ACP Journal Club 2005;142:46.

108. Topol EJ, Falk GW. A coxib a day won't keep the doctor away. [comment]. Lancet 2004;364:665-74.

CHAPTER 31 – THE CLINICAL LABORATORY IN RHEUMATOLOGY

1. McCarty DJ, Kohn NN, Faires JS. The significance of calcium pyrophosphate crystals in the synovial fluid of arthritic patients: the "pseudogout syndrome". Ann Intern Med 1962;56:711-37.
2. McCarty DJ, Hollander JL. Identification of urate crystals in gouty synovial fluid. Ann Intern Med 1961;54:452-60.
3. Hasselbacher P. Arthrocentesis, synovial fluid analysis, and synovial biopsy. In: Klippel J, Weyand CM, Wortmann RL eds. Primer on the Rheumatic Diseases, 11th ed. Atlanta GA: The Arthritis Foundation 1997; 98-104.
4. Shmerling RH, Delbanco TL. The rheumatoid factor: an analysis of clinical utility. Am J Med 1991;91:528-34.
5. Wolfe F, Cathey MA, Roberts FK. The latex test revisited. Rheumatoid factor testing in 8,287 rheumatic disease patients. Arthritis & Rheum 1991;34:951-60.
6. Litwin D, Singer JM. Studies of the incidence and significance of antigamma globulin factors in the aging. Arthritis Rheum 1965;8:538-80.
7. Homburger HA. Cascade testing for autoantibodies in connective tissue diseases. Mayo Clin Proc 1995;70:183-4.
8. Barland P, Lipstein E. Selection and use of laboratory tests in the rheumatic diseases. Am J Med 1996;100(2A):16S-23S.
9. Kallenberg CG, Wouda AA, The TH. Systemic involvement and immunologic findings in patients presenting with Raynaud's phenomenon. Am J Med 1980;69:675-80.
10. Lee DM, Shur PH. Clinical utility of the anti-CCP assay in patients with rheumatic diseases. Annals of the Rheumatic Diseases 2003;62:870-4.
11. Conner GE, Nelson D, Wisniewolski R, et al. Protein antigens of the RNA-protein complexes detected by anti-SM and anti-RNP antibodies found in serum of patients with systemic lupus erythematosus and related disorders. J Exp Med 1982;156:1475-85.
12. Reichlin M. Autoantibodies to the Ro RNP particles [editorial]. Clinical & Experimental Immunology 1995;99:7-9.
13. Buyon JP, Winchester RJ, Slade SG, et al. Identification of mothers at risk for congenital heart block and other neonatal lupus syndromes in their children. Comparison of enzyme-linked immunosorbent assay and immunoblot for measurement of anti-SS-A/Ro and anti-SS-B/La antibodies. Arthritis Rheum 1993;36:1263-73.
14. Powell FC, Winkelmann RK, Venencie-Lemarchand F, et al. The anticentromere antibody: disease specificity and clinical significance. Mayo Clin Proc 1984;59:700-6.
15. Steen VD, Powell DL, Medsger TA, Jr. Clinical correlations and prognosis based on serum autoantibodies in patients with systemic sclerosis. Arthritis Rheum 1988;31:196-203.
16. Miller FW. Myositis-specific autoantibodies. Touchstones for understanding the inflammatory myopathies [clinical conference]. JAMA 1993;270:1846-9.
17. Rao JK, Weinberger M, Oddone EZ, et al. The role of antineutrophil cytoplasmic antibody (c-ANCA) testing in the diagnosis of Wegener granulomatosis. A literature review and meta-analysis. Ann Intern Med 1995;123:925-32.
18. Kallenberg CG, Brouwer E, Weening JJ, Tervaert JW. Anti-neutrophil cytoplasmic antibodies: current diagnostic and pathophysiological potential. Kidney Int 1994;46:1-15.

19. Choi HK, Merkel PA, Walker AM, Niles JL. Drug-associated antineutrophil cytoplasmic antibody-positive vasculitis: prevalence among patients with high titers of antimyeloperoxidase antibodies. Arthritis Rheum 2000;43:405-13.
20. Harris EN. Syndrome of the black swan. Br J Rheumatol 1987;26:324-6.
21. Roubey RA. Autoantibodies to phospholipid-binding plasma proteins: a new view of lupus anticoagulants and other "antiphospholipid" autoantibodies. Blood 1994;84:2854-67.
22. Thiagarajan P, Pengo V, Shapiro SS. The use of the dilute Russell viper venom time for the diagnosis of lupus anticoagulants. Blood 1986;68:869-74.
23. Hebert LA, Cosio FG, Neff JC. Diagnostic significance of hypocomplementemia [editorial]. Kidney Int 1991;39:811-21.
24. Atkinson JP. Complement deficiency. Predisposing factor to autoimmune syndromes. Am J Med 1988;85:45-7.
25. Sox HC Jr., Liang MH. The erythrocyte sedimentation rate. Guidelines for rational use. Ann Intern Med 1986;104:515-23.
26. Kanik KS, Bridgeford PH, Germain BF. Polymyalgia rheumatica with a low erythrocyte sedimentation rate: Comparison of 10 cases with 10 cases with high erythrocyte sedimentation rate. J Clin Rheumatol 1997;3:319-323.
27. Bull BS, Westengard JC, Farr M, et al. Efficacy of tests used to monitor rheumatoid arthritis. Lancet 1989;2(8669):965-7.
28. Salvarani C, Cantini F, Boiardi L, Hunder GG. Polymyalgia rheumatica and giant-cell arteritis. New England Journal of Medicine 2002;347:261-71.
29. Visser M, Bouter LM, McQuillan GM, et al. Elevated C-reactive protein levels in overweight and obese adults. JAMA 1999;282:2131-5.
30. Hull SK, Collins LJ. Clinical inquiries. How useful is high-sensitivity CRP as a risk factor for coronary artery disease?. Journal of Family Practice 2005;54:268, 271-2.
31. Brout JC, Clauvel JP, Danon F, et al.Biologic and clinical significance of cryoglobulins. A report of 86 cases. Am J Med 1974;57:775-88.
32. Ferri C, Greco F, Longombardo G, et al. Antibodies to hepatitis C virus in patients with mixed cryoglobulinemia. Arthritis Rheum 1991;34:1606-10.
33. Khan MA, Khan MK. Diagnostic value of HLA-B27 testing in ankylosing spondylitis and Reiter's syndrome. Ann Intern Med 1982;96:70-6.
34. Weyand CM, Hicok KC, Conn DL, Goronzy JJ. The influence of HLA-DRB1 genes on disease severity in rheumatoid arthritis. Ann Intern Med 1992;117:801-6.
35. Cid MC, Ercilla G, Vilaseca J, et al. Polymyalgia rheumatica: a syndrome associated with HLA-DR4 antigen. Arthritis Rheuma 1988;31:678-82.
36. Chajek-Shaul T, Pisanty S, Knobler H, et al. HLA-B51 may serve as an immunogenetic marker for a subgroup of patients with Behçet's syndrome. Am J Med 1987;83:666-72.
37. Delmas PD. Clinical use of biochemical markers of bone remodeling in osteoporosis. Bone 1992;13(Suppl 1):S17-21.

ACKNOWLEDGEMENTS

The following figures have been reproduced with kind permission of Merit Publishing International, *Visual Diagnosis self-tests on Rheumatology, 2nd Edition.*

Chapter 1 : Figs 1, 2, 4, 3, 5
Chapter 2 : Figs 1, 2, 3, 4, 5
Chapter 7 : Figs 2,3,4,5,6
Chapter 8 : Fig 1
Chapter 12: Fig 2
Chapter 15: Figs 2, 3, 4

Chapter 17: Figs 1, 2
Chapter 18: Figs 3,4
Chapter 28: Fig 1
Chapter 29: Fig 1

The following figures have been reproduced with kind permission of The European League against Rheumatism. Website http://www.eular.org

Chapter 9: Fig 1
Chapter 11: Fig 1
Chapter 12: Figs 1, 3
Chapter 14: Figs 1
Chapter 15: Fig 1
Chapter 17 Fig 3
Chapter 18: Figs 1, 2, 5, 6, 7, 8
Chapter 19: Fig 1
Chapter 20: Figs 1,2, 3, 4
Chapter 27: Figs 1, 2
Chapter 30: Fig 1
Chapter 31: Fig 1
Chapter 32: Fig 1

INDEX

A

B

C

D

G

H

I

J

K

L

M

N

S

T

NOTES